Affirm * Confirm * Claim Your Life!

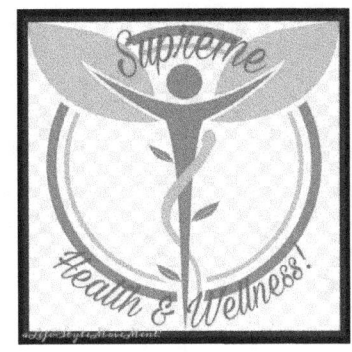

Affirm * Confirm * Claim Your Life!

Writing YOUR Own Book of Healing, Health & Abundant Life!

| Supreme Health Staff & Scientist | Kareem Tyree Khalil Malik | Gabriella Monique |

Supreme Health & Fitness!   Knowledge Of Self Series Vol 2!

*Affirm * Confirm * Claim Your Life!*

Affirm * Confirm * Claim Your Life!

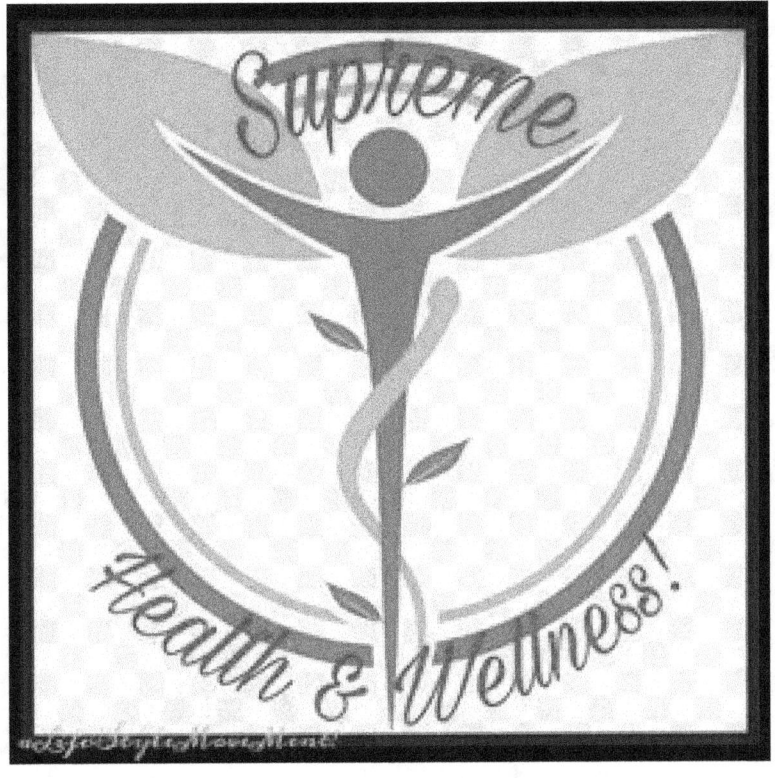

Supreme Health and Fitness by Sean Ali!

Achieving and Maintaining Supreme Health and Fitness by Increasing the Level of Knowledge and Science of Life!

A LifeStlye MoveMent!

Affirm * Confirm * Claim Your Life!

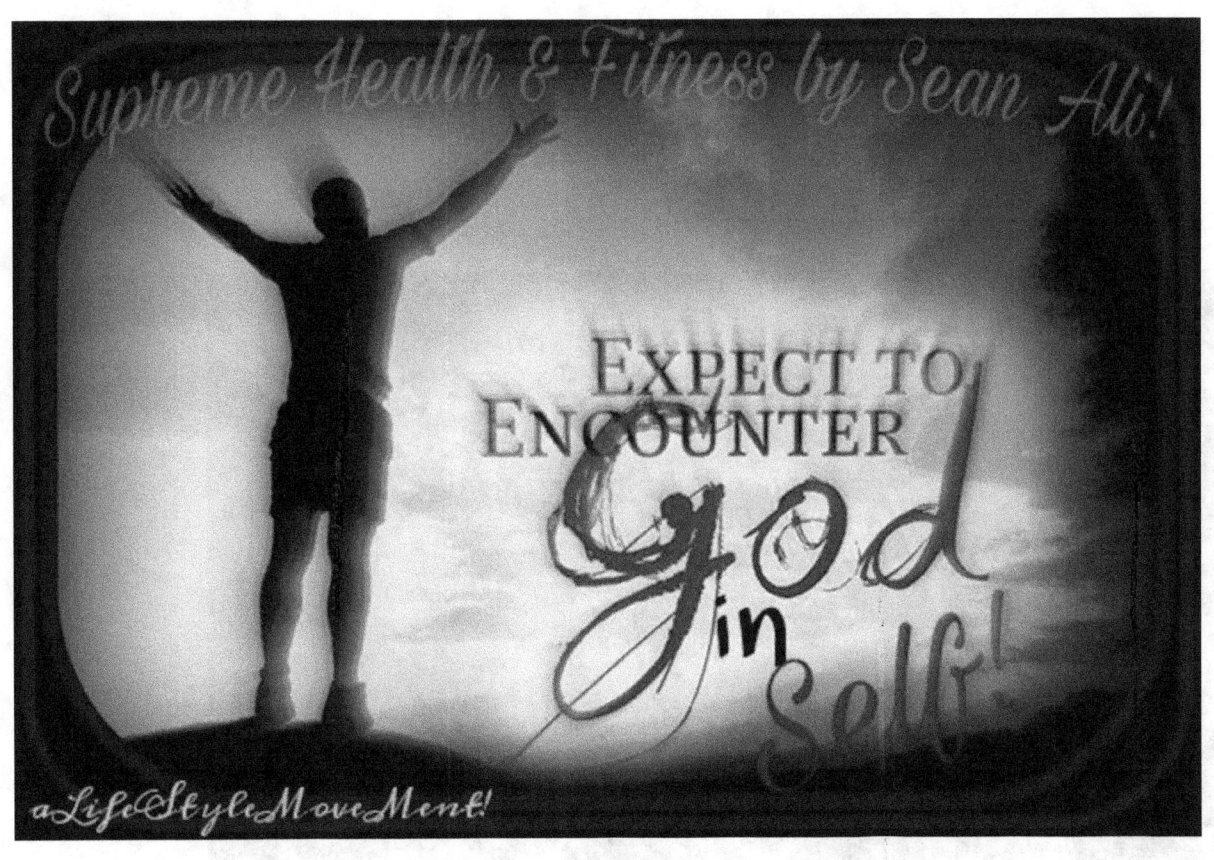

*Affirm * Confirm * Claim Your Life!*

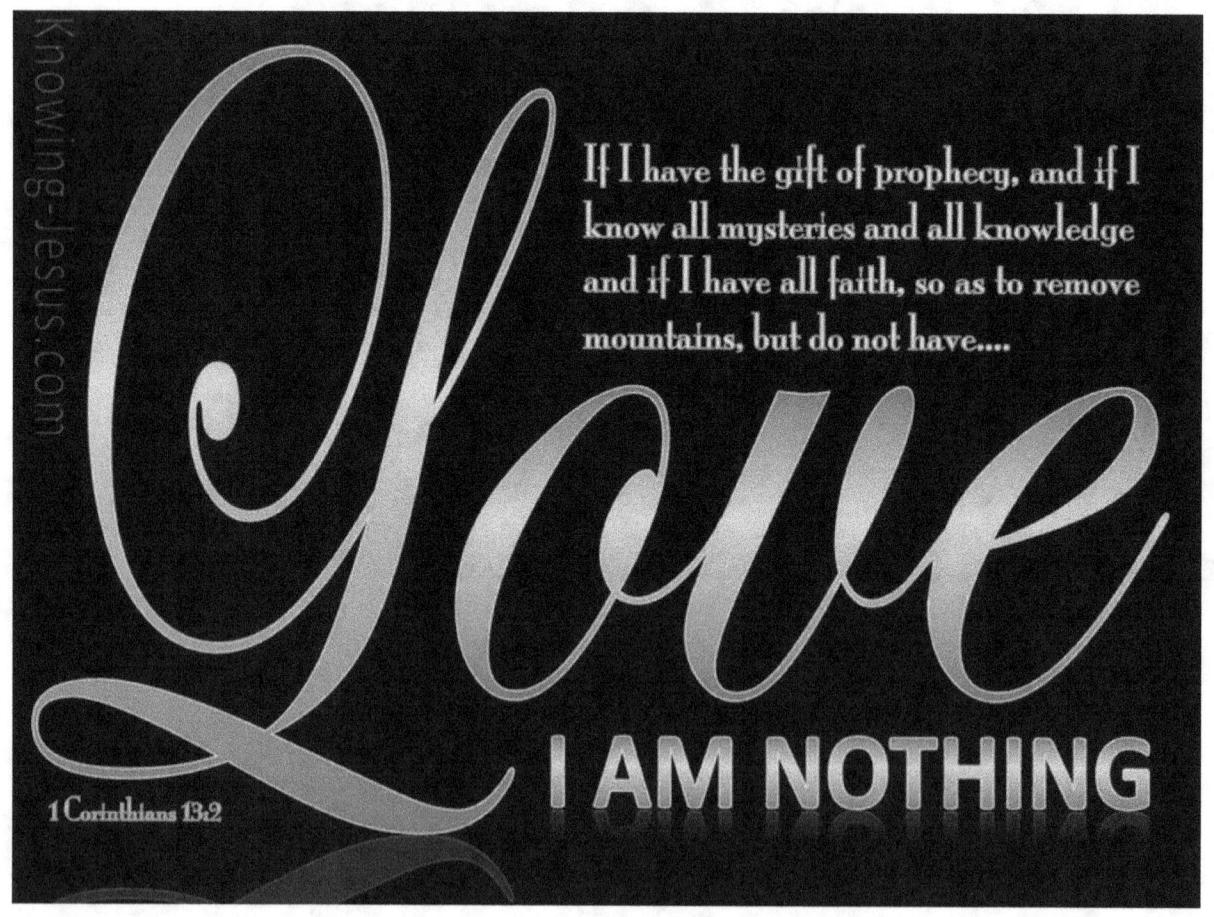

Affirm * Confirm * Claim Your Life!

Table of Contents

Introduction ...   ... Page 11

Chapter One ... Intentionally Learning Self ...   ... Page 23

Chapter Two ... Develop Your Critical Thinking ...   ... Page 35

Chapter Three ... Understanding Critical Writing ...   ... Page 45

Chapter Four ... Understanding Critical Reading ...   ... Page 51

    *Your Self Assessment ...   ... Page 57

    *Who Am I Activity ...   ... Page 58

    *Self Awareness Test ...   ... Page 59

    *Life Satisfaction Activity ...   ... Page 60

    *Self Esteem Check-Up ...   ... Page 61

    *Goals & Dreams Activity ...   ... Page 62

    *How I Feel Activity ...   ... Page 63

    *Building Confidence Activity ...   ... Page 64

    *Self Awareness Activity ...   ... Page 65

Affirm * Confirm * Claim Your Life!

Chapter Five ... Understanding Self Concept ... ... Page 67

    *All About ME Activity ... ... Page 70

    *Self Esteem Worksheet ... ... Page 74

    *How Can I Improve Self Activity ... ... Page 75

Chapter Six ... Guidelines – Improving Self-Concept ... ... Page 77

    *Self Esteem Journal ... ... Page 86

    *Support System ... ... Page 87

    *Positive Expression of Self ... ... Page 88

Chapter Seven ... Mastering Self Perception ... ... Page 89

    *Emotional Intelligence Activity ... ... Page 105

    *Self Talk Worksheet ... ... Page 107

Affirm ... ... Page 109

    *Improve Your Moment Activity ... ... Page 117

    *5 Things I Like About Self ... ... Page 118

    *Life Story Activity ... ... Page 119

I AM Statements ... ... Page 122

Affirm * Confirm * Claim Your Life!

I Can Statements …	… Page 125
I Will Statements …	… Page 127
* Self Love Worksheet …	… Page 133
Confirm …	… Page 137
You Are Statements …	… Page 144
You Will Be Statements …	… Page 147
Chapter Eight … Poewer of Words …	… Page 149
*Gratitude Journal …	… Page 154
*Respect Worksheet …	… Page 155
*Open To Create Activity …	… Page 159
Chapter Nine … Developing Your Creativity …	… Page 161
Chapter Ten … Guidelines – Improving Perception …	… Page 167
Claim …	… Page 175
I Claim Statements …	… Page 177
*Emotional Intelligence Activity ,,,	… Page 152

Affirm * Confirm * Claim Your Life!

*Mind, Body & Spirit Activity ... ... Page 183

Chapter Eleven ... Understanding FEAR ... ... Page 185

*Challenging Negative Thoughts Activity ... ... Page 191

*Not To Do List ... ... Page 192

*Stress Diary ... ... Page 193

*Time Mangement Activity ... . Page 195

Chapter Twelve ... Achievement Motivation ... ... Page 197

Conclusion ... ... Page 207

Resources and References ...

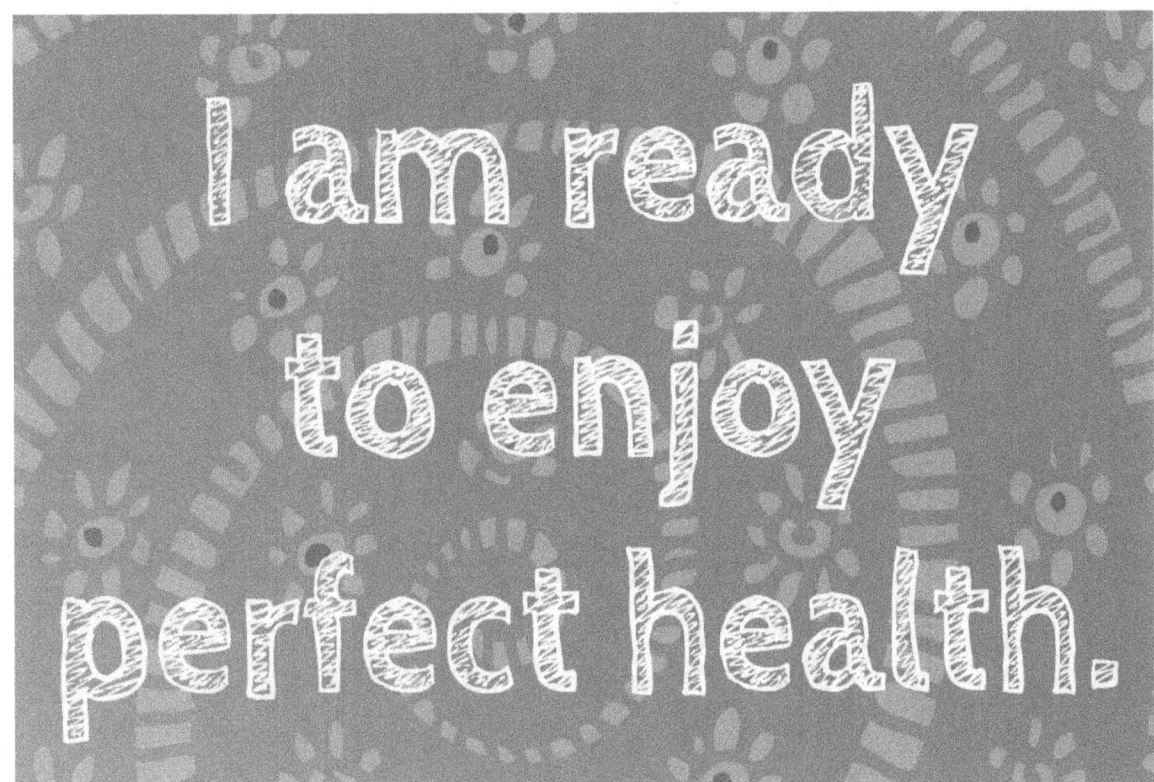

*Affirm * Confirm * Claim Your Life!*

Affirm * Confirm * Claim Your Life!

Introduction!

* * * * *

Peace and Blessings of Health!

This small book represents Volume 2 of the Knowledge of Self Series and is the accompanying Work-Book to my Exciting and Ground-Breaking 1st Volume – Science of Thought & Art of Thinking! In this Exciting Volume we use activities to expound on and apply the Principles and Scientific concepts to use the Art of Thinking to Create our own Healing, Health, Life & Power, with the main focus centered right on YOU ..... this is because the ONLY Person that can Heal and Empower YOU – IS YOU!!!!

The only thing a Health care professional can do I to help YOU create the proper Healthy environment in YOU that allows YOUR Body to HEAL ITSELF ... Just as THE CREATOR Created it to do!

Although our Physical Body I created with the necessary Elements to heal itself, the Bai of Healing IS WITHIN OUR MIND!!

Affirm * Confirm * Claim Your Life!

So, the Purpose of this book is to lay the Foundation of Mental and Spiritual Healing by Building the Will and Strengthening and Increasing Mental Power with Written and Physical Activities.

There are only 3 Very EAY Step, NO WRONG Answer and Absolute SUCCESS .... YOU WILL GET BACK EACTLY 100% OF WHAT YOU PUT IN!!!!

You will be writing Your own Great Story of Excellence, Power, Health and Love that will help u to successfully carry You into the Enjoyment of Abundant Life!!!!

In this book, we explore the science of Emotion, the science of Thinking, the science of Language and the science of ACTION and how they relate to the 3 Principles of the book – AFFIRM, CONFIRM & CLAIM!!!

The Science of Affirm, Confirm and Claim is based on the concepts of Writing and Reading YOUR Own Healing, Health, Life and POWER!

Some of what we want to accomplish with this volume includes creating a new Definition of ourselves – based on HOW we see ourselves instead of others. We also want to accomplish Intentional Learning about ourselves. Unfortunately, many of us don not know ourselves and can only define ourselves according to how others define us.

Affirm * Confirm * Claim Your Life!

In this Volume are some of the sciences of Intentional Learning and I use some of the principles so that we can Intentionally Learn about ourselves and how we can use them to Develop and Cultivate our Healing, Health, Life and Power!

We explore Perceptions and the science of the Perception process. By understanding the process of perception, we can correct any imbalance or defects in our perception skills.

We become able to use our own perception to create our own Image and Understanding of WHO WE ARE!

We use our own perception to create our own Healing, Health, Life and Power!

We can use our own perception to become an Intentional Learner of Ourselves!

Included in this Volume are several activities and exercises that you can use to create or build on your Self-Awareness, that will help you build and increase your Self-Perception and that will help you understand and over-come any FEARS or mis-conceptions that you may have developed about yourself.

The beginning stage of developing YOUR Mind-Set of Power is the stage of Affirm and consists of Thinking and then Writing 'I AM' statements.

Affirm * Confirm * Claim Your Life!

You THINK of the "I AM" statements which requires you to spend 30 Minutes of Focused and Devoted THINKING of YOU!

Not just any type of Thoughts, but the Highest Quality Thoughts – Thoughts that are based on creating the Environment of Healing, Health, Life and Power. Many of us have never attempted to Focus and Devote our Thinking on our own Healing and Health, which is the underlying factor of WHY we get sick and can't heal.

Examples of Thinking these 'I AM' statements are You Mentally picturing your image and health and creating statements like: I AM Healing! I AM Beautiful! I AM Strong! I AM Intelligent!

Words have Electrical and Chemical Actions that correspond to their Meaning and Use. So, during this stage you Think of and apply to yourself the Highest Quality and Power words. As you Think of them, the Electrical Energy/Current of these words is being created IN YOU!

The corresponding Chemical Hormones of the words are being transported throughout your body. You are beginning the process of creating Healing, Health, Life and Power IN YOURSELF!

After producing these thoughts, you are now ready to transform your Un-Seen Thoughts INTO a Seen Reality!

Affirm * Confirm * Claim Your Life!

Now you take Action by WRITING these same 'I AM' statements that you previously thought of yourself. Writing is Action. Physical Action.

In order for your muscles to Move an electrical impulse is created that causes your muscles to contract = Motion.

We have Motion the we can Cause - Voluntary and we have Reflex Motion or Involuntary motion, that our body causes on its own.

By Writing your "I AM" statements, you are creating a Determined and Focused Electrical Current to Move yourself.

Your body begins to coordinate Motion, which is the physical expression of your un-seen Thought. Similar to how you produce Movement from the thought of eating to complete the Act of eating to satisfy a hunger craving. In this case, you are using your Thought to produce the Actins that Causes your Healing, Health, Life and Power by first Thinking, then Causing Motion of yourself on Healing, Health, Life and Power words, ideas and emotions.

This created Electrical Energy further reinforces the Electrical and Chemical Energy you originally created in you from Thinking these statements. You INCREASE Building Your HEALING, Your HEALTH, Your LIFE and Your POWER!

Affirm * Confirm * Claim Your Life!

The Act of Writing about Your own Healing, Health, Life and Power creates the environment where you BECOME that which you are Writing!

The second stage is CONFIRM. In the Confirm stage we are further converting our Thoughts into ACTION and simultaneously increasing the changes of Self into our Healing, Health, Life and Power.

With Confirm, we actively TELL ourselves the written 'I AM' statements. The progression is evolved from our un-seen Thought which we make manifest into Reality by transferring it into Written form.

Next, we increase and build on this by Speaking into Existence that which we wrote. In doing so we are activating and utilizing 3 of our 5 Senses – Touch, Sight and Hearing!

As a Man Thinketh – So IS he!

In this stage, you actively Talk to yourself. You LOOK at your reflection and you communicate with yourself in the 3rd person and reinforce your 'I AM' statements.

Example: Sean, You ARE Healing!   Sean, You ARE Beautiful!   Sean, You ARE Intelligent!   Sean, You ARE Strong!

Affirm * Confirm * Claim Your Life!

While doing this, you are activating and engaging your Sense of Sight – Seeing Yourself SAY these empowering statements of stimuli.

You are engaging your Hearing – Hearing statements of Healing, Health, Life and Power BEAT into your eardrum and immediately impacting your Brain, Mind and Thoughts. Your Ears are connected directly to your Brain!

You are Confirming your Healing, Health, Life and Power by speaking into existence your own Story – Produced from your own Thoughts.

This is your Book of Life! We all need inspiration from time to time. So, instead of using another person's story for Inspiration or Motivation – you can Open Your Own Book and draw Inspiration, Motivation and Power from YOURSELF!!!!!

CLAIM IS THE ACTION STAGE…… YOU LIVE THAT WHICH YOU HAVE WRITTEN AND SPOKEN YOURSELF TO BE!

CLAIM YOUR HEALING!

CLAIM YOUR HEALTH

CLAIM YOUR LIFE!

*Affirm * Confirm * Claim Your Life!*

CLAIM YOUR POWER AND GO BE GREAT!!!

Open this book and begin the process of Writing Your Own story of Your Healing, Your Health, Your Life and Your Power!!!!!

Your Healing, Your Power and Your Greatness is already in You, with this book, we want to help You to SEE it and have the ability to Successfully make Your Healing, Your Life and Your Power manifest!!!

PEACE!

Sean Ali

Supreme Health & Fitness!

*Affirm * Confirm * Claim Your Life!*

hi!
today will be...
awesome

daily goal
desired outcome

phone calls	email	media

Supreme Health & Fitness!   *Knowledge Of Self Series Vol 2!*

*Affirm * Confirm * Claim Your Life!*

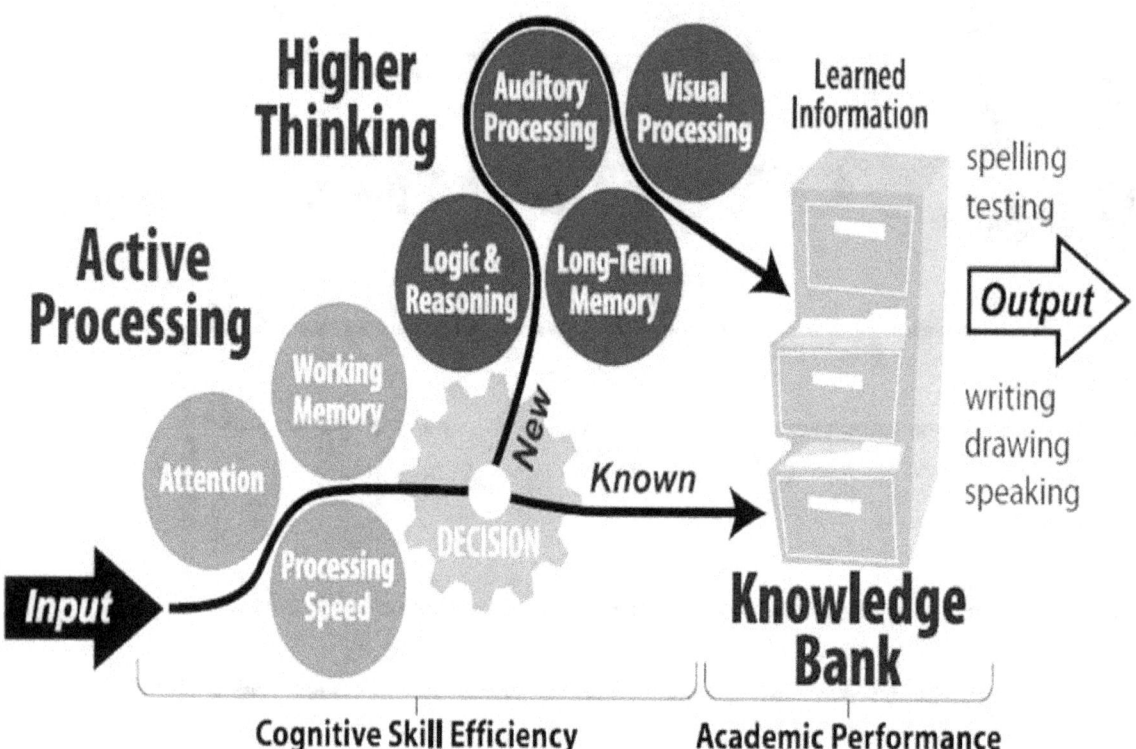

The Learning Model illustrated here helps point out the difference between the processing functions of Active Processing and Higher Thinking Systems on the left and the storage and distribution function of the Knowledge Bank on the right. All new or unfamiliar information must be processed before it is useful in life, work, or academic performance. Strong, efficient cognitive skills are essential to successful learning.

Active Processing
- Always active and running
- Automatically handles most information that is taken in
- Needs to be fast and efficient
- Some information can't be automatically processed

Higher Thinking
- Mental skills are used to process new information
- Solves problem when tasks aren't automatically processed
- General thinking ability
- Determines how well information is stored and retained

Knowledge Bank
- Learned information and data
- Different from mental processing skills
- Storage must grow as one matures
- Size and use are dependent upon processing abilities

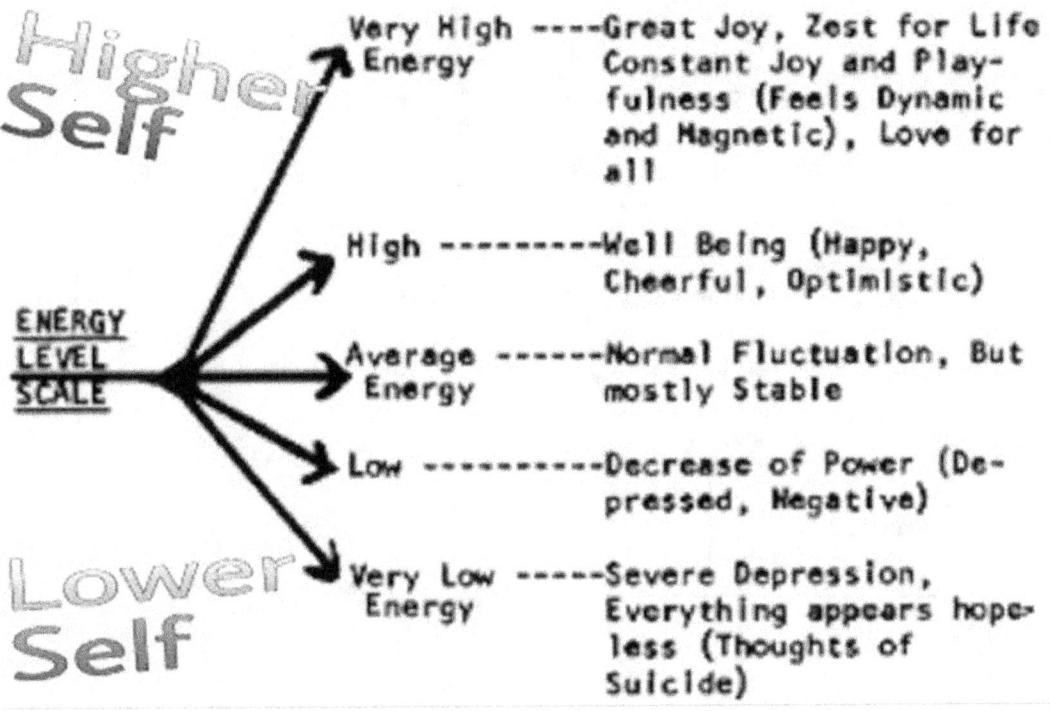

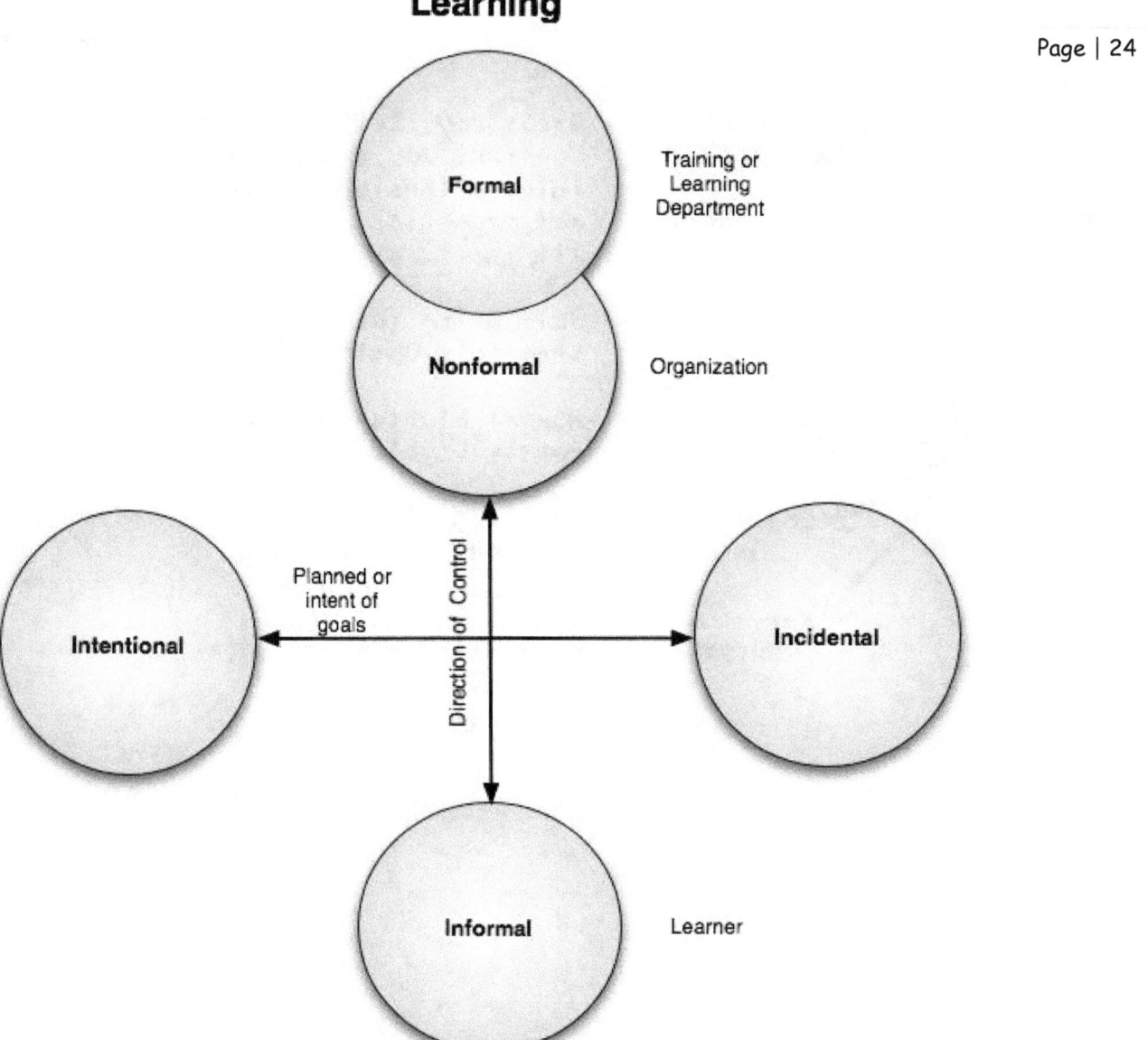

Chapter One

Intentionally Learning Your Self

* * * * *

The requirements of learning have changed significantly over the past one hundred years. Where once learning to memorize large amounts of information was the mark of a successful student, today having the knowledge, skills, and judgment to select and use data accurately, interact with others appropriately, and use new technologies efficiently are important for student success.

Today you are required to **learn how to learn**—that is, move what is outside your head to inside your mind, working with it by reading critically and writing critically, studying and owning it, and then presenting your newfound knowledge, understanding, and insights for discussion, feedback, and refinement.

How Do We Learn?

What is learning, and what are some basic forms of learning?

Learning is the process of acquiring new and relatively enduring information or behaviors. In **Associative Learning**, we learn that certain events occur together. In classical conditioning, we learn to associate two or more stimuli (a *stimulus* is any event or situation that evokes a response). In operant conditioning, we learn to associate a response and its consequences.

Through **Cognitive Learning**, we acquire mental information that guides our behavior. For example, in observational learning, we learn new behaviors by observing events and watching others.

Through **Intentional Learning**, we Direct and Focus our Energy to become Successful.

*Affirm * Confirm * Claim Your Life!*

With this chapter we will explore the best concepts of Learning to use them to Learn About Ourselves! Knowledge IS Power …. The MORE you KNOW about yourself = The MORE Power and Control you can manifest over and on yourself.

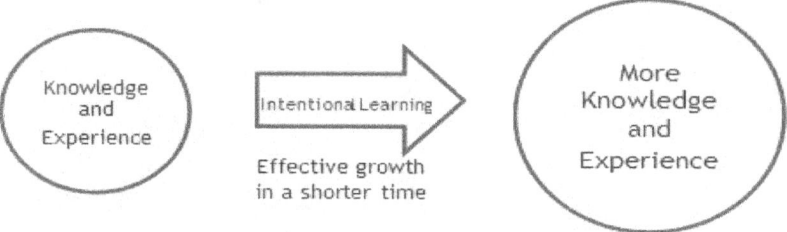

Learning By Observation

What is observational learning, and how do some scientists believe it is enabled by mirror neurons?

In *observational learning,* as we observe and imitate others we learn to anticipate a behavior's consequences because we experience vicarious reinforcement or vicarious punishment. Our brain's frontal lobes have a demonstrated ability to mirror the activity of another's brain. (Some psychologists believe *mirror* neurons enable this process.) The same areas fire when we perform certain actions (such as responding to pain or moving our mouth to form words) as when we observe someone else performing those actions.

What is the impact of prosocial modeling and of antisocial modeling?

Children tend to imitate what a model does and says, whether the behavior being *modeled* is *prosocial* (positive, constructive, and helpful) or antisocial. If a model's actions and words are inconsistent, children may imitate the hypocrisy they observe.

Self-Regulation

This is the ability to consciously examine your own thoughts and behavior, to identify which of them is causing you to be unproductive, and to determine alternative thoughts and behaviors that will lead you to a successful learning outcome.

Self-regulation is steeped in self-discipline—a type of self-discipline that is not rigid but flexible, one that is open to facing reality, aimed at problem solving, and prepared to redirect your energy toward achieving your goal.

As Marzano (1992) notes, self-regulation involves the discipline and focus to:

1. Be aware of your own thinking.
2. Plan and then monitor your use of time.
3. Evaluate the effectiveness of your actions.
4. Be open to feedback.

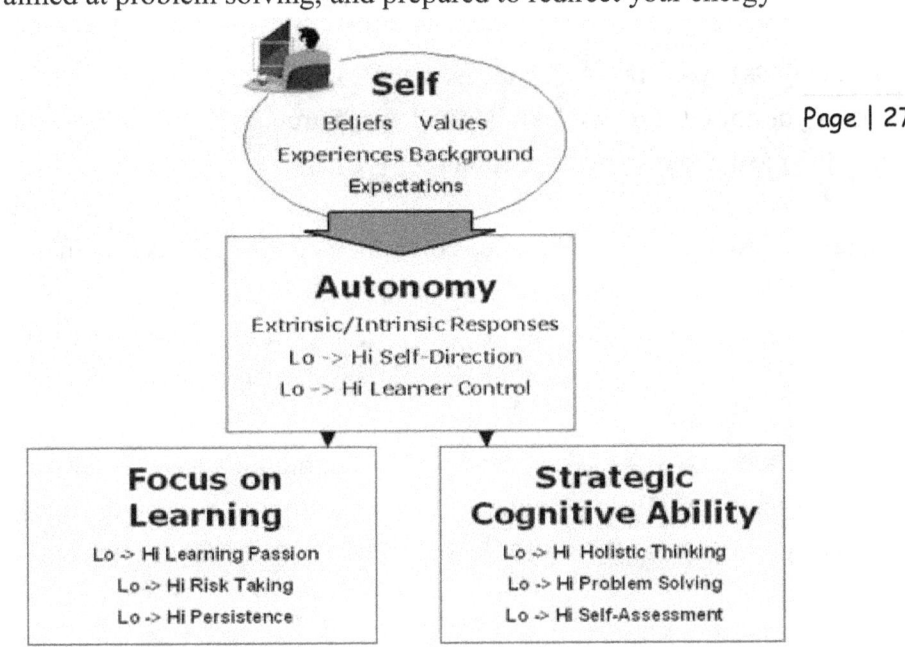

Metacognition

The pathway to becoming an intentional learner begins with noticing, understanding, and regulating your thoughts and behavior before, during, and after a learning experience.

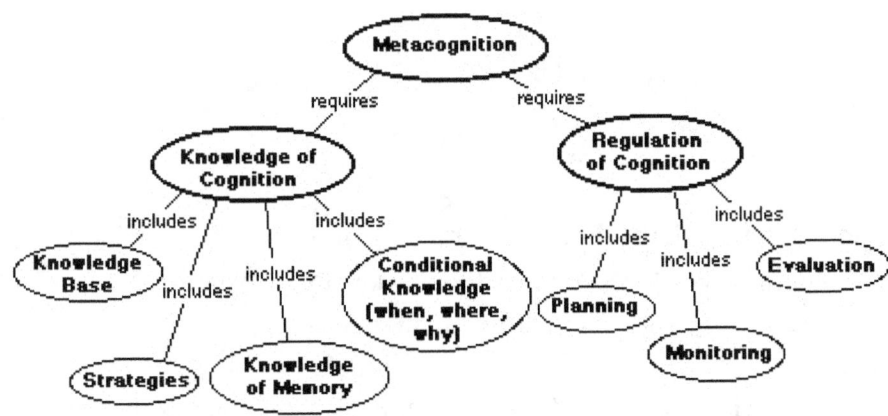

This learning behavior is known as metacognition, which lies at the heart of intentional learning. It consists of the phases your mind goes through as you are seeking to learn.

As you metacognate, you are moving the external happenings of the world to the internal operations of your mind. You are taking in the world around you, making sense of it, and developing the means to respond appropriately.

In the context of intentional learning, metacognition is defined as the internal talk that goes on within your mind as you are learning. While its traditional definition is "thinking about thinking," the pioneers of metacognitive study described it more specifically as "learning to direct one's own mental processes with the aid of words" (Vygotsky, 1986, p. 108).

Your internal talk consists of the "chatter" of your Learning Patterns as they call to one another—expressing their feelings, concerns, or the actions they want to engage in. Each of your Patterns plays an important role in your learning; each has a different perspective; and each has a distinct voice.

Learning Process

Most of the learning is incidental. Some of it is intentional.

- ***Intentional*** - *learning acquired as a result of a careful search for information.*

- ***Incidental*** - *learning acquired by accident or without much effort.*

The communication among your Learning Patterns forms your metacognition. Rather than being a distraction, the chatter among your Patterns allows you to actively listen to how your Patterns are at work within your mind, pulling and tugging you in different directions.

This awareness provides you with the insight necessary for "purposeful decision-making about how to proceed with the task" (Baird, Fensham, Gunston, & White, 1991, p. 164).

*Affirm * Confirm * Claim Your Life!*

Self-regulation allows you to take charge of your Patterns and "talk back" to them, employing strategies that help you complete the task you have been given.

We will examine the 4 Learning Patterns and apply the principles to becoming a successful Intentional Learner of ourselves!

4 Learning Patterns

Sequence

The learner who uses Sequence first typically begins a learning task by asking, "What are the directions?" "What am I expected to do?" "Can you post some examples for me to look at? I don't want to start until I know what your expectations are."

Those who use Sequence at a high level want the security of seeing what the project is expected to look like. They want to make certain there is no hidden agenda.

If you use Sequence at a high level, Your security—your sense of self as a learner—comes with "I can do this well by using the techniques that have brought me success before. I will use them over and over." If you use Sequence to a high degree, you thrive on practice and enjoy checking with others to see how they are approaching the task.

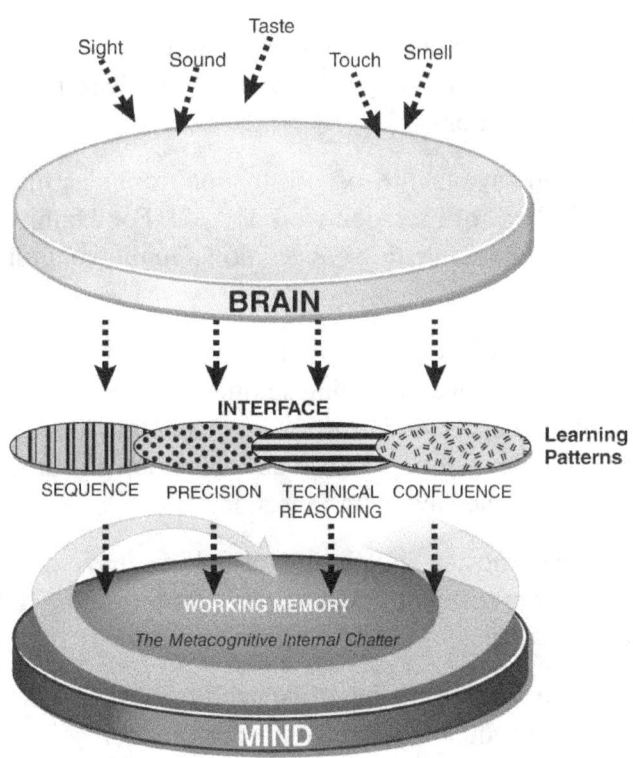

However, if you avoid Sequence, you often skip over reading and following directions, consciously choose not to live by a schedule, and rarely double-check your work. You allow yourself to miss deadlines often or don't complete the task as assigned.

Avoiding Sequence can make completing work on time feel like an annoyance. It can entice you into believing that you don't need to read or follow directions. In fact, directions remain a mystery to you, since your mind does not easily wrap itself around a set of written or spoken directions.

This principle is important when establishing how to Learn Self. Becoming an Intentional Learner of Self does require a few guidelines.

Affirm * Confirm * Claim Your Life!

Precision

If you use Precision first, you want to receive thorough explanations, ask lots of questions, and be correct. You typically begin an assignment by gathering a lot of data, a lot of facts, and a lot of specifics. You can be relentless in seeking information.

You may be labeled a "walking encyclopedia," and you probably love trivia—sports stats, game shows, etc. When your Precision is Use First level, you may enjoy taking a test because it allows you to measure how much you know and understand about a specific topic.

One hazard of Use First Precision is that you do not always use your time wisely because you think you can squeeze in one more text message, one more check of your Facebook status, one more detail. Those who use Precision first need information, act with precision, and feel good when the work is done exactingly.

Of course, not everyone uses Precision to the same degree and in fact, you may actually avoid Precision. If you avoid it, you rarely read for pleasure, don't attend to details, and tune out long-winded conversations.

With the ready availability of information from electronic search engines, you can make even your Avoid level of Precision work for you. For example, you can more quickly skim and scan information without getting bogged down in the voluminous amount of information you have found.

On the other hand, you might find the amount of information available to you overwhelming. You may turn instead to reading summaries and abstracts (when appropriate to your research) instead of reading extensive articles. As long as the source you have selected is factually based and logically developed, you can use abbreviated sources to make your case and thereby succeed, even when avoiding Precision.

When developing a new definition of Self, we have to go in-depth and think about Self on many levels and from many different angles – ranging from mental, spiritual, physical, business, pleasure and social.

You will use the information of yourself to complete the learning of yourself and knowing what type of learner you are before you begin can increase your chance of Success!

Technical Reasoning

Technical Reasoning is very different from Precision in the way it operates within your mind. While Precision is the Pattern of the most words, Technical Reasoning is the Pattern of the fewest words. In fact, its most unique trait is that it allows you to think without words.

Affirm * Confirm * Claim Your Life!

The downside is that if you use Technical Reasoning first you may struggle to find the right words to articulate your thoughts. First and foremost, you look for relevance and practicality. You live to fix things and solve problems, and you prefer to work by yourself.

When you use Technical Reasoning first you understand tools, gadgets, and technical instruments. You speak their language. You think in operational terms. You like to take things apart to see what makes them tick and put them back together without any leftover screws.

Interestingly, the Pattern of the most words, Precision, and the Pattern of the fewest words, Technical Reasoning, can work together at the Use First level. However, Technical Reasoning typically affects working relationships by limiting the amount and flow of information provided by Precision, keeping it to the minimal "need to know." Only relevant facts are shared with coworkers and "information for information's sake" is not.

A lot of people are Technical learners and to think of yourself and about yourself is a strong point of those with this learning style. you are literally taking yourself apart – piece by piece of all the outside definitions given to you by others so that you can re-build with your own definitions.

Confluence

Has anyone ever told you that you think outside the box? Don't color inside the lines? This is Confluence at work. You thrive on change. You see the jointedness rather than the disjointedness of life. Confluence can lead you, in the middle of a focused activity, to say something totally unrelated, and the response you hear is, "Where did that come from?" It came from within you. Perhaps you saw something on television, or in a movie, or in a book, and now in the middle of your conversation you see a connection—one that others might not see. As one highly Confluent preschooler explained when asked the source of her comment during a class discussion: "It just came out of nowhere."

When Confluence is your Use First level, you use metaphors. Rather than taking the time to select the precise words needed to explain something in detail, you liken the new piece of information to something that in your mind is very similar. By using a metaphor, you have a quick way to explain what you are seeing or experiencing without having to take the time to express it with exactness. Using a metaphor allows you to paint a broad stroke comparison in a very Confluent manner.

The key to using the Pattern of Confluence effectively is to anchor your ideas and your excitement about them to a plan, well researched information, or a well-grounded purpose. In this way you can use your Confluence with intention to achieve a specific outcome.

Affirm * Confirm * Claim Your Life!

When connected to your entire team of Learning Patterns, Confluence can provide the spark to move you to greater innovation and achievement. It all depends upon your intentional use of all of your Patterns.

Of course, if you avoid Confluence, you think taking risks is foolish and wasteful. You are cautious in how you go about making life decisions. You would rather not make mistakes, especially if your avoidance of Confluence is tied to using Precision first.

To go in-depth and study self we literally have to think outside the box. The BOX is the definitions of others that we have used to define and see ourselves as.

To form our own definitions, we have to remove the old and one of the best ways to do that is with the Confluence style of learning.

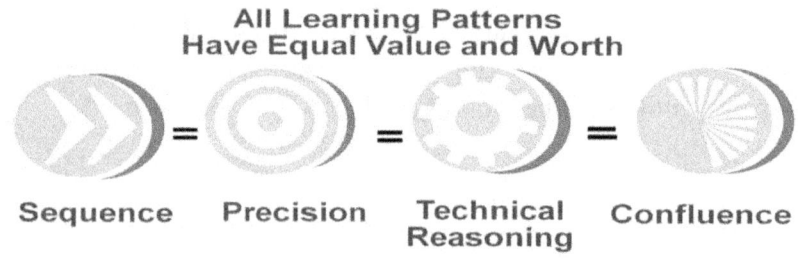

Patterns do not work in isolation. You are never only one Pattern. Your Pattern combination always consists of all four Patterns working as a team.

Your Patterns act in concert with each other to create wholeness—a dynamic for success. Working as a team of mental processes, they form a vibrant relationship that you can feel at work in you and that others can observe readily.

Most importantly, your Patterns are your Patterns. There is no combination of Patterns that is stronger; there is no combination of Patterns that is weaker. Your Patterns are who you are. They are right for you.

They work well for you—when you know how to use them with intention.

Understanding how your Learning Patterns affect your learning behavior is central to becoming an intentional learner. At the heart of intentional learning is the awareness that you know how to self-regulate the use of your learning processes.

Key to self-regulation is your awareness that avoiding any Pattern allows your other Patterns to dominate how you respond to the world around you.

Affirm * Confirm * Claim Your Life!

Without a conscious effort on your part to know and use each of your Patterns with intention, they can keep you from responding appropriately to situations—and in doing so, can keep you from being a successful learner.

Only when you listen to your internal metacognitive chatter can you begin to take charge and respond appropriately to it. You may often miss the voice of your metacognition because you are surrounded by other audible distractions: ringtones, people's voices, digitized music.

Or you may ignore the chatter because you have decided not to notice it. One reason you might opt to ignore your internal talk is because you are not prepared to listen to its message.

Your metacognition consists of a quartet of voices: Sequence, Precision, Technical Reasoning, and Confluence. It challenges you to make sense of their message and to hear more than the harmony and disharmony within your thinking; it forces you to listen and make defining decisions. That is not easy to do when your Patterns are arguing about how to proceed or how to achieve. Listening to your metacognition takes practice, patience, and skill.

Sequence		Precision	
alphabetize	list	calibrate	label
arrange	order	detail	measure
bullet(ed)	organize	describe	name
classify	pros and cons	document	record (facts)
compare and contrast	put in a series	examine	observe
develop	put in order	explain	perform accurately
distribute	review	identify	specify
format	sequence		
frame (structure)	show an array		
group	show an example		

Technical Reasoning		Confluence	
assemble	fix	act carefree	improvise
build	implement	brainstorm	innovate
construct	just do it	chance	invent
demonstrate	operate concretely	concoct	make-up
engineer	problem solve	create	originate
erect	represent graphically	dream-up	risk
experience	write briefly	imagine	take a chance
figure out			

*Affirm * Confirm * Claim Your Life!*

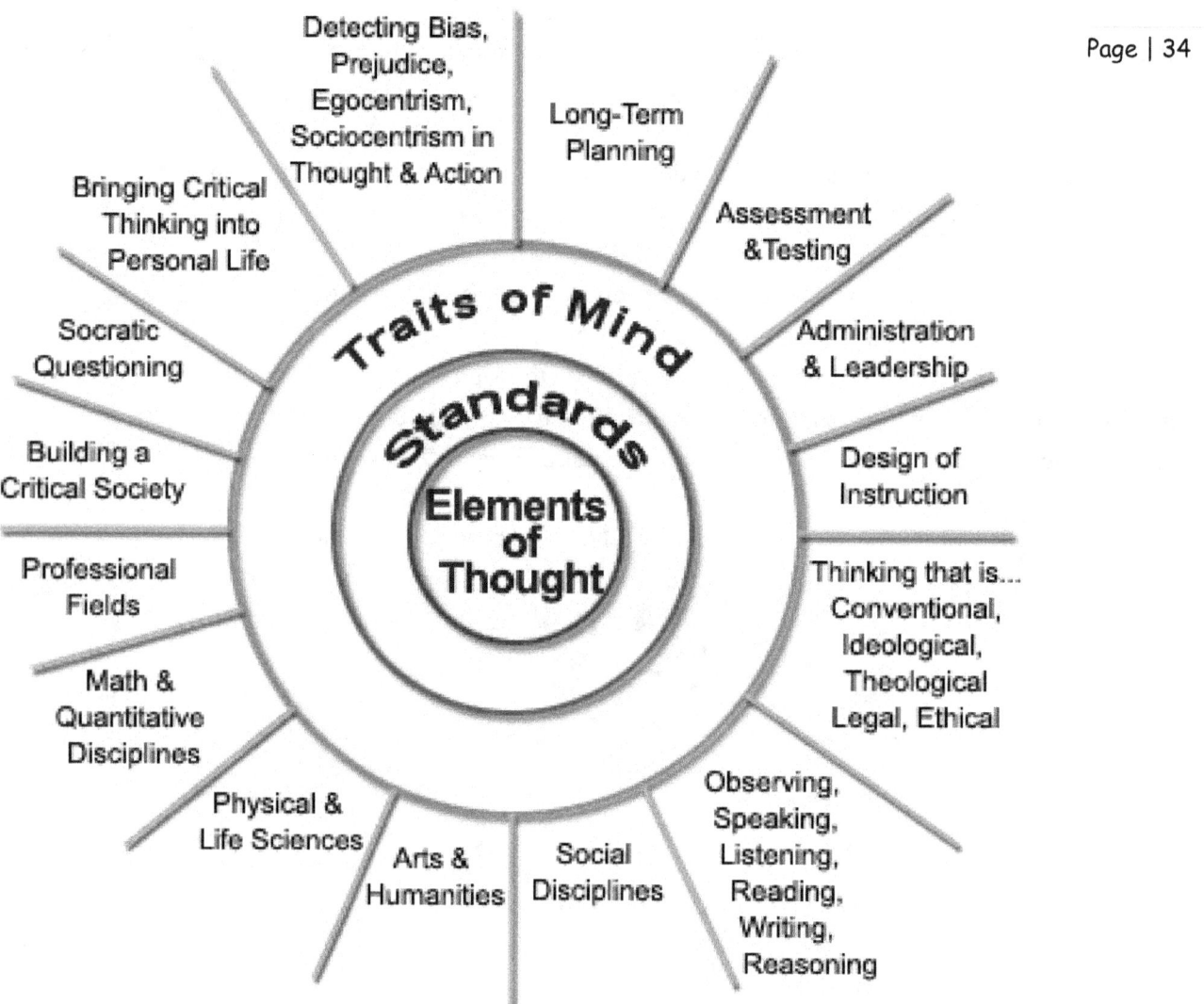

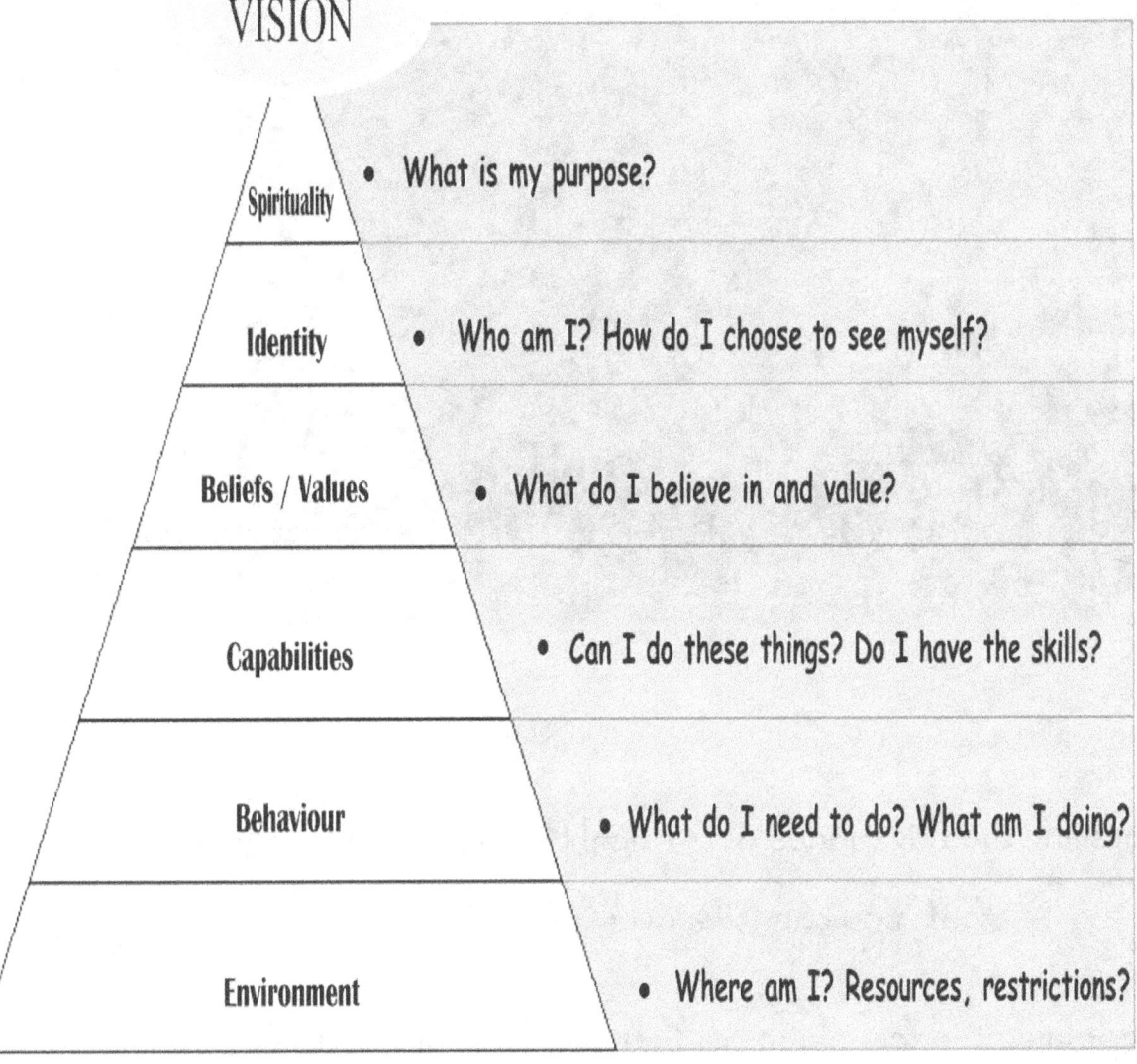

*Affirm * Confirm * Claim Your Life!*

Critical Reading & Thinking

- Critical *reading* is a technique for **discovering** information and ideas within a text.
- Critical *thinking* is a technique for **evaluating** information and ideas, for deciding what to accept and believe.
- Critical *reading* refers to a careful, active, reflective, analytic reading.
- Critical *thinking* involves reflecting on the validity of what you have read in light of the prior knowledge and understanding.

You are applying the techniques of Critical Reading on YourSelf so that You can Discover YOU!

You are applyibg the techniques of Critical Thinking so that You can Actively and Analytically Re-Deifne YOU!

Chapter Two

Developing Your Critical Thinking Skills

*****

The Skills of Critical thinking does not occur by luck or by chance. You are not born a critical thinker. The skills and behaviors that produce critical thinking develop over time and through experience.

Whether you develop your Critical Thinking Skills and the Depth of them depth and scope of your abilities are solely dependent upon YOU!

Your Critical thinking skills improve when you intentionally practice them.

Critical thinking

- Critical thinking is the cornerstone of one's ability to function in today's society. According to Scriven & Paul (n.d.),
- it...can be seen as having two components:
  - a set of skills to process and generate information and beliefs, and
  - the habit, based on intellectual commitment, of using those skills to guide behavior.

While there are many sophisticated definitions of critical thinking, they are frequently so abstract that they do not connect with you or your life. For now, let's define critical thinking as an intentional act by you, the learner, to ask questions, to use reasoning, and to gather facts in order to arrive at an accurate, logical conclusion.

Criteria for Critical Thinking

1. It must be reasonable as opposed to arbitrary or unreasonable.

Critical thinking must rely on the use of valid supporting evidence and appropriate inference from which, in general, the best conclusions are drawn.

2. Critical thinkers must be reflective.

They must consciously evaluate their own and others' thinking in an effort to improve it.

3. Critical thinking is focused thinking.

It is thinking with a purpose. That purpose is to make the best decision about what to believe or do.

One way to look at critical thinking is as a type of mental gymnastics/exercise by which you strengthen your thinking and enhance your learning stamina. In this case you are Strengthening and Enhancing Your Learning of YOURSELF!

The following list of learning "actions" helps define, in specific behaviors, what it means to be thinking, reading, and writing critically about yourself and why doing so is essential to succeeding in creating YOUR Healing, Health, Life and Power.

Note that at the end of each sentence are the Learning Patterns strategic to each action:

1. Develop your knowledge by thoughtfully questioning (use Precision and Confluence).
2. Read for deep meaning (use Precision and Technical Reasoning).
3. Base your opinions on facts and weigh information in the balance (use Sequence and Precision).
4. Examine your logic and reasoning when forming your conclusions about yourself (use Sequence, Precision, and Technical Reasoning).

Cognitive neuroscience is the study of mental brain processes and its underlying neural systems. This includes thinking and behavior and is underpinned by the learning brain. Therefore, cognitive neuroscience looks at how the brain learns, stores, and uses the information it acquires.

It is through learning that the brain enables us to adapt to our ever-changing environment.

*Affirm * Confirm * Claim Your Life!*

The area of overlap between different disciplines, including cognitive neuroscience and education, has been identified as a transdisciplinary field of study called educational neuroscience or neuroeducation.

According to The Royal Society February 2011 report, *The Brain Waves Module 2: Neuroscience: Implications for Education and Lifelong Learning,* this field investigates basic biological processes involved in becoming literate and numerate, and explores learning to learn, cognitive control, flexibility, and motivation, as well as social and emotional experiences.

Why is Critical Thinking Important?

- To learn is to think.
- To think poorly is to learn poorly.
- To think well is to learn well.
- All content, to be learned, must be intellectually constructed.
- Memorizing **IS NOT** learning.

Our Brain and Learning

Learning is a physical process in which new knowledge is represented by new brain cell connections. The strength and formation of these connections are facilitated by chemicals in the brain called growth factors.

We now know from neuroscience that the availability of these growth factors can be enhanced. For example, specific exercise routines, optimal sleep structure, and silencing the mind can all enhance the availability of these growth factors.

Both Nature and Nurture affect the learning brain. People have different genetic predispositions, but experience continuously shapes our brain structure and modifies behavior.

During the past decade numerous peer-reviewed publications have connected the fields of neuroscience with education and learning. Several studies report structural and functional changes in the brain related to training.

*Affirm * Confirm * Claim Your Life!*

A working understanding of how the brain learns and performs is an invaluable new skill. It is essential for the future success of Your Healing, Health, Life and manisfestation of YOUR POWER!

We intuitively understand the need to acquire new knowledge, which optimizes the value of Self. What is less obvious, but of great importance, is that creative and innovative thinking processes in our brains are built on the foundation of knowledge.

Our brains continuously draw on this knowledge base to create simple solutions to complex problems. Knowledge provides the building blocks for innovation, which is the number one priority for Your Success!

Active engagement is necessary for learning

Changes in neural connections, which are fundamental for learning to take place in the brain, do not seem to occur when learning experiences are not active. Many research studies suggest that active engagement is a prerequisite for changes in the brain.

Not surprisingly, just listening to a presentation or lecture will not lead to learning. Powerful training initiatives that stimulate active engagement include facilitation, simulation, games, and role play.

All learning has an emotional base

Neuroscientists believe that emotions are fundamental to learning. One of the earlier advocates of this was Plato, who mentioned more than 2,000 years ago that "All learning has an emotional base."

Motivation in the brain is driven by emotion. Individuals are motivated to engage in situations with an emotionally positive valence and avoid those with an emotionally negative valence.

What better emotional motivation can we have then of the one attached to Healing ourselves?

Research findings indicate that different aspects of memory are activated in different emotional contexts, and that demonstrates there are links between emotion and cognition.

Training professionals can design learning sessions that tap into the emotions. This is the Foundational Principle of this book!

You are Training specifically and purposefully to create Your Own Healing!

You are Training with the explicit focus of creating Your Own Power!

Affirm * Confirm * Claim Your Life!

Focused attention is fundamental to acquiring new knowledge

We now have learned from neuroscience that sustained focus is largely an unconscious process but essential for learning and creative thinking.

Actively silencing the mind through a process of focused attention (focusing on the major senses while breathing deeply) or open monitoring (actively allowing incoming stimuli without reacting or responding to it) for 20 minutes per day will go a long way toward enhancing the ability for focused and sustained attention.

Therefore, it is a powerful imperative to include time for meditation and breathing in the design of classroom programs.

Deployment of short learning sessions will increase knowledge retention

The brain remembers the first part and the last part of a training initiative best. This is called the primacy-recency effect.

The middle period of learning should be filled with the least important information, and shorter learning sessions will reduce the middle "down" period.

This is why training sessions ideally should be no more than 20 minutes, with planned "brain breaks" separating sessions.

In this workbook, we introduce you to 'short' activities that are easier to assimilate and apply!

Use learning techniques that enhance memory formation

Learning techniques that have shown to enhance memory formation include elaborating, verbalizing, writing and drawing, and sharing learned information during and at the end of a learning session.

Interweaving different subject matter categories during a training event enhances the learning process.

So, in this workbook, you will be Thinking, Writing and Reading.

You will be examining your Emotional, Mental and Physical Wellness!

Simply, this means that three different subjects can be learned by studying them simultaneously, moving from one subject to the next in an open-ended interweaving fashion.

That is because the brain learns and packages new knowledge even while we are not aware of it; it's a continuous and vastly unconscious process. The brain continues to learn and consolidate new knowledge unconsciously, even as we consciously start to focus on new material.

Use it or lose it

The adult brain changes following the acquisition of new skills. However, the changes in the brain reverse when people do not have the opportunity to use the skills they have developed.

Unfortunately, many training initiatives are less effective because people can't apply their learning in the workplace after completion of training.

This is one of the benefits of this particular learning. It provides on-demand learning and knowledge that can be reviewed at any time and any place.

When you need inspiration or motivation – all you have to do is open and read your own story of Healing, Life, Power and of YOUR GREATNESS!!!!!

Multitasking slows down learning

Multitasking has become a way of living and working for many people. Unfortunately, our brains are not wired for multitasking because most of us can only apply our full conscious attention to one stimulus at a time. (A small proportion of the population, called "super-taskers," can pay attention to two stimuli at one time.)

Our working memory—this is the part of the brain that allows us to focus our attention on a task such as reading—continues to interact with our long-term memory where we retrieve and store specific information.

If we try to conduct two tasks at the same time, we must switch between the different tasks and an overload results between our working memory and long-term memory, which causes us to lose time.

Multitasking is not effective and costs an estimate of $650 billion because employees spend one-third of their time interrupting existing tasks to continue later with the same tasks.

Therefore, it is important during training programs to limit multitasking. With this workbook, you have a SINGLE task – Re-Define and Create Yourself according to YOU!!

In doing this, you will develop and build your Power over yourself to facilitate Your Healing, Your Health, Your Power and Your Greatness!!!!

Affirm * Confirm * Claim Your Life!

Remember, Your Body Moves and Does what YOU TELL IT TO DO!!!!!!

By, learning yourself, you gain Mastery over Self. In this Mastery you gain the ability and knowledge to direct your body to Heal itself!

You direct YOUR Body to manifest its Power and IT WILL!!!!!

Enhancing brain performance capacity supports learning

Though learning preferences differ from person to person, all human brains function in the same general way. Understanding how your brain absorbs and stores new information can help you optimize your performance.

Practice Leads To Stronger Connections IN Your Brain

When it comes to creating stronger, faster connections in the brain, practicing the skill or information that you wish to fully master is essential.

This is because regular practice — whether it involves reading a history textbook, listening to a science podcast or solving a calculus problem — causes your dendrites to grow thicker and to coat themselves with a fatty layer.

With enough practice, these thickened brain fibers will eventually form double connections to one another.

When this occurs, signals carrying information can travel faster to and from different parts of your brain. The fatty coating on brain fibers also speeds up your brain's ability to process information. Brain fibers with double connections are very strong and enduring.

Thus, continually practicing a given skill to acquire information or ability can help solidify that information or ability in your brain more permanently.

As you are Practicing your Healing ... Your Brain and Body becomes permanently attuned to Healing!

As you are Practicing Your Power .... Your Brain and Body becomes permanently attuned to POWER!!!

Affirm * Confirm * Claim Your Life!

Type of Practice Directly Impacts what You Learn

It is important to remember that the brain grows fibers that relate to what you are practicing.

With this workbook, You will be Growing the Brain Fibers associated with and Needed for to create the environment for Your Healing!

You will be creating the Brain Fibers Needed to make manifest Your POWER!!!!

You will be Growing the Brain Fibers You Need to BE GREAT!!!!

This fact is especially important to keep in mind if you are enrolled in courses that require hands-on skills, such as calculus, chemistry, physics and studio art.

In such classes, it's essential to not just listen to and watch how to perform a specific skill, but to also perform that skill yourself. This will help you truly learn it.

Barriers to Critical Thinking

- **Egocentricity and resistance to change.** Change can threaten our identity, our security, our sense of self-worth. Alternative viewpoints may force us to admit we were wrong, which is often difficult.
- *Arrogance and ignorance go hand in hand.*
- **Wishful thinking and self deception.** How we want things to be may influence how we see them, what evidence we select, and what we choose to ignore. Superstitions are often maintained in this way.

*Affirm * Confirm * Claim Your Life!*

CRITICAL THINKING SKILLS

1 **Knowledge** *Identification and recall of information*	define fill in the blank list identify	label locate match memorize	name recall spell	state tell underline
	Who _____? What _____? Where _____? When _____?		How _____? Describe _____. What is _____?	
2 **Comprehension** *Organization and selection of facts and ideas*	convert describe explain	interpret paraphrase put in order	restate retell in your own words rewrite	summarize trace translate
	Re-tell _____ in your own words. What is the main idea of _____?		What differences exist between _____? Can you write a brief outline?	
3 **Application** *Use of facts, rules, and principles*	apply compute conclude construct	demonstrate determine draw find out	give an example illustrate make operate	show solve state a rule or principle use
	How is _____ an example of _____? How is _____ related to _____? Why is _____ significant?		Do you know of another instance where _____? Could this have happened in _____?	
4 **Analysis** *Separating a whole into component parts*	analyze categorize classify compare	contrast debate deduct determine the factors	diagram differentiate dissect distinguish	examine infer specify
	What are the parts or features of _____? Classify _____ according to _____. Outline/diagram/web/map _____.		How does _____ compare/contrast with _____? What evidence can you present for _____?	
5 **Synthesis** *Combining ideas to form a new whole*	change combine compose construct create design	find an unusual way formulate generate invent originate plan	predict pretend produce rearrange reconstruct reorganize	revise suggest suppose visualize write
	What would you predict/infer from _____? What ideas can you add to _____? How would you create/design a new _____?		What solutions would you suggest for _____? What might happen if you combined _____ with _____?	
6 **Evaluation** *Developing opinions, judgements, or decisions*	appraise choose compare conclude	decide defend evaluate give your opinion	judge justify prioritize rank	rate select support value
	Do you agree that _____? Explain. What do you think about _____? What is most important?		Prioritize _____ according to _____? How would you decide about _____? What criteria would you use to assess _____?	

Critical reflection

Critical reflection analyzes experience by exploring social, political, educational, and cultural contexts and exposing the assumptions that dictate response.

Critical reflection enables us
- to engage in transformative learning by engaging both reason and emotion (Taylor, 2001);
- to situate ourselves within a broader social context;
- to understand our values, beliefs, and biases;
- to work through seemingly contradictory feelings, reactions, and understandings in order to better work with clients;
- to assess our learning so that our learning informs our practice.

- **Assumption analysis** – challenging our beliefs and social structures in order to determine their impact on our practice;
- **Contextual awareness** – determining the social and cultural contexts that influence our assumptions;
- **Imaginative speculation** – imagining alternative ways of thinking in order to challenge our current ways of thinking;
- **Reflective skepticism** – questioning universal claims or unexamined interactions by suspending or temporarily rejecting previous knowledge about the subject.

*Affirm * Confirm * Claim Your Life!*

Chapter Three
Understanding Critical Writing

*****

Critical writing depends upon your cognitive processes performing myriad tasks with remarkable speed. The main task, simply stated, is to communicate from the inside out by having the mind convert its internal thoughts to external expression (Johnston, 2005). Needless to say, critical writing can be challenging skill. It requires your language processing "muscles" to be "flexed" regularly, so they are ready to do some "heavy lifting" to place words in clear, logical, persuasive order—just like you need to keep real muscles strong to be able to move and lift objects as needed. It takes practice, and the more you do it, the better you get.

Critical writing takes many forms (short answers, paragraph responses, postings, essays, research papers). Regardless of the required format, gathering your thoughts from inside your mind and presenting them for public view can be the most challenging and, in some cases, the most agonizing of human acts.

For the purposes of this book we will be exercising the Critical Writing Skills on ourselves!

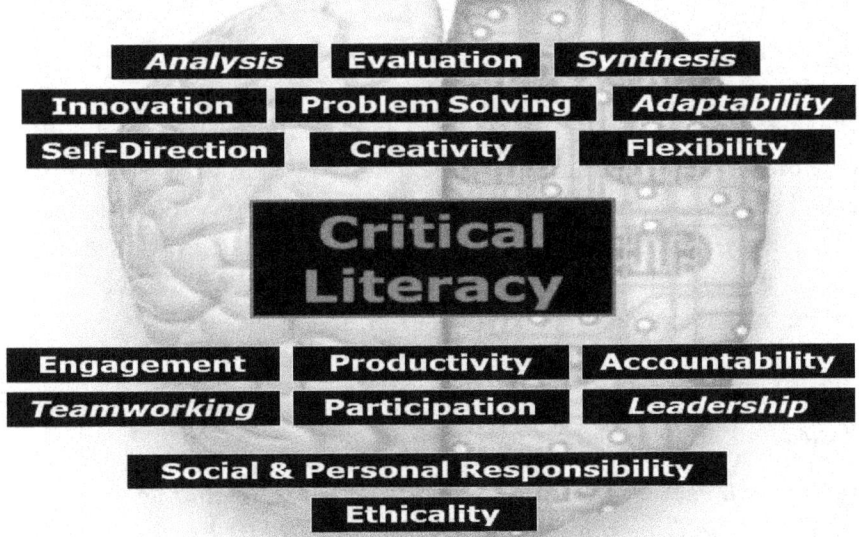

Affirm * Confirm * Claim Your Life!

The following depicts in words what the writing process involves in terms of the brain-mind connection:

When you write you are
recording,
expressing,
articulating,

communicating your
thoughts
feelings
experiences
ideas in

symbolic representation by consistently using
lines scratched on paper or
symbols digitally relayed from a keyboard to a screen
that have the same meaning each time they are viewed by the human eye and

translated by the brain's neuro-receptors and
interpreted, and either
immediately relayed to the recipient or

stored by the working memory for
retrieval and
expression
at the appropriate time. (Johnston, 2005)

Writing for Your Audience - YOU

Everything is written for an audience, and for a specific purpose. The instructions that come with your iPad are written for you, the owner, and their purpose is to explain to you how to load it with your favorite applications and get the most out of your new toy. Shakespeare wrote Hamlet for his Elizabethan-era audience, and for future generations of playgoers, and his purpose was to entertain his audience and expose it to profound ideas about human nature. When you leave a note for someone, you write it with the person in mind and for a specific purpose.

In this book, you are writing for the express specific purpose of YOU!

You are Writing words with Your Healing in Mind!

You are Writing specific words that will create the environment in Your MIND that will increase the Power You have over Yourself and allow You to HEAL YOURSELF!!

*Affirm * Confirm * Claim Your Life!*

You will be Writing for the audience of yourself to BECOME POWERFUL!

You will Write the Words that will create the Foundation for You to Successfully Enjoy Your Abundant Life!

Using Your Learning Patterns to Master Critical Writing

Critical writing, like critical reading, relies on the development of intentional skills. One way to learn the skill of critical writing is to read the work of other writers and to use their methods as models to follow.

Understand how you learn and then read about the experiences of others similar to yourself, so you can identify how to deploy their strategies in order to improve your writing.

Hints for Writers Who Are Short on Confluence and Long on Sequence

Here are a few tips to help Sequence users get started writing—and keep going:

Picture a hotel desk bell on your workstation. Now pick up a pen and start brainstorming ideas for that project you're avoiding. Every time you allow thoughts of "That will never work," or "What will that look like?" or "We've done that before," ding that bell. Write every idea down. Don't stifle your creativity by censoring yourself. One idea leads to another. You may not invent something, but you surely can tweak an existing idea or concept.

You must get past the idea that you need an opening paragraph in order to begin. Essays and reports can be written in sections, and not necessarily in order. Start in the middle. Come back to the beginning and write an introduction once your main points are down on paper. Eventually you will see your argument or story as a whole, but for the time being, be willing to develop sections as they unfold in your mind. Afterward you can put them in the order that makes the story or the argument flow and add the introduction and conclusion.

Most important of all is to write free of the rules that keep you grounded and stuck.

Write.

Get your thoughts down first; then pay attention to spelling and punctuation, verb tense, and exact wording.

Write into existence Your HEALING!!!!!

Write into existence Your POWER!!!

Write into existence Your GREATNESS!!!!

Universal Design for Learning

Recognition Networks
The "what" of learning

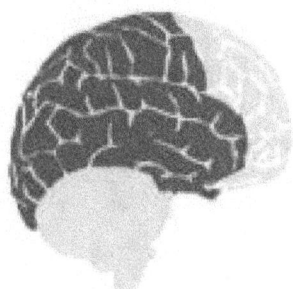

How we gather facts and categorize what we see, hear, and read. Identifying letters, words, or an author's style are recognition tasks.

 Present information and content in different ways

More ways to provide Multiple Means of Representation

Strategic Networks
The "how" of learning

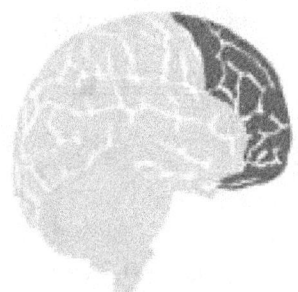

Planning and performing tasks. How we organize and express our ideas. Writing an essay or solving a math problem are strategic tasks.

☑ Differentiate the ways that students can express what they know

More ways to provide Multiple Means of Action and Expression

Affective Networks
The "why" of learning

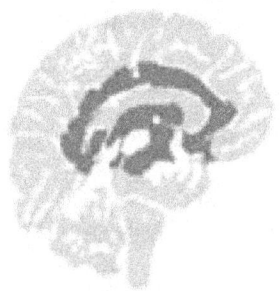

How learners get engaged and stay motivated. How they are challenged, excited, or interested. These are affective dimensions.

 Stimulate interest and motivation for learning

More ways to provide Multiple Means of Engagement

Affirm * Confirm * Claim Your Life!

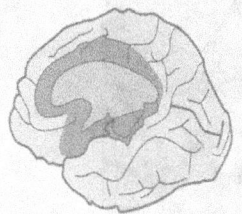

AFFECTIVE NETWORKS:
THE **WHY** OF LEARNING

Engagement

For purposeful, motivated learners, stimulate interest and motivation for learning.

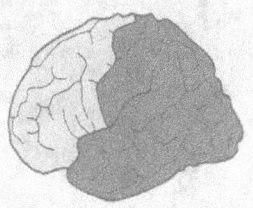

RECOGNITION NETWORKS:
THE **WHAT** OF LEARNING

Representation

For resourceful, knowledgeable learners, present information and content in different ways.

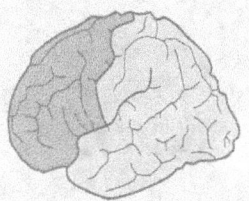

STRATEGIC NETWORKS:
THE **HOW** OF LEARNING

Action & Expression

For strategic, goal-directed learners, differentiate the ways that students can express what they know.

Critical Reading & Critical Thinking

- **Critical reading**: technique for discovering information & ideas
  > careful, active, reflective, analytical reading

- **Critical thinking**: technique for evaluating information & ideas
  > reflecting on validity in light of prior reading and understanding of the world

*Affirm * Confirm * Claim Your Life!*

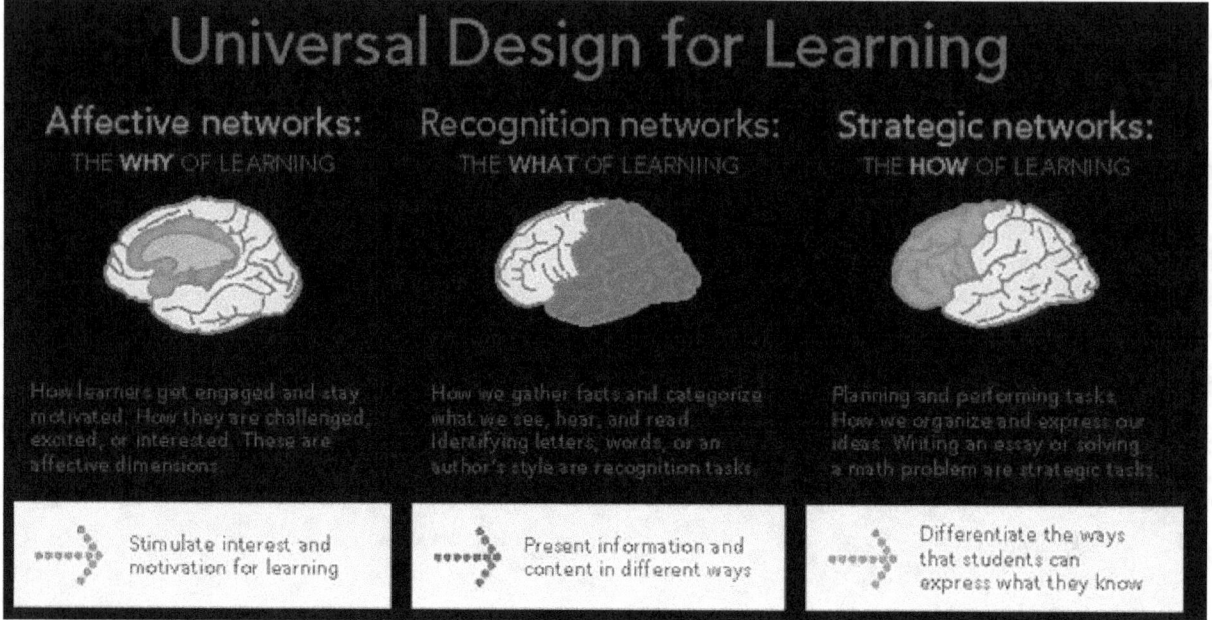

Characteristics of Critical Readers

- They are honest with themselves.
- They resist manipulation.
- They overcome confusion.
- They ask questions.
- They base judgments on evidence.
- They look for connections between subjects.
- They are intellectually independent.

Affirm * Confirm * Claim Your Life!

Chapter Four
Understanding Critical Reading
*****

While the ability to read refers to an individual's ability to translate letters into words, and words into a message, critical reading requires that the reader drill down into the intention of the writer in order to discern the thoughts, ideas, feelings, and message the writer sought to convey.

The critical reader sees words as more than a group of letters but as a container of thought to be mined for deep meaning.

Have you ever thought of your words or sentences as containers?

You can create your own containers for yourself and fill them with Healing, Health, Life and Power letters/words.

Consider that words are thoughts packaged and transported through the container of language. The famous urban sociologist and historian Lewis Mumford named human language as the single most influential container used by mankind (Mumford, 1968).

Mumford believed that language is mankind's universal container of thoughts, feelings, ideas, and records. Its invention allowed individuals to control many aspects of their lives and equipped them to transport thoughts contained in systems of symbols (languages) from one place to another.

- "Critical" is not intended to have a negative meaning in the context of "critical reading."
- Definition: An active approach to reading that involves an in depth examination of the text. Memorization and understanding of the text is achieved. Additionally, the text is broken down into its components and examined critically in order to achieve a meaningful understanding of the material.

*Affirm * Confirm * Claim Your Life!*

The first, and most important, container of language is human memory. Once that container could no longer hold all the information needed, the container for storing language manifested in the forms of sand tablets, plant fibers, animal skins, and, centuries later, microchips.

The language of spoken and written words is not the only language, however. Mathematics is its own unique language; Braille and sign language, likewise.

Whatever the container used, it is only as powerful as the human mind that can open the container and decode the message. Reading performs this action (Wolf, 2009, p. 9).

Reading opens the container of language and releases the expression stored within it. Since YOU filled these containers, when YOU OPEN them YOU GET YOUR HEALING, HEALTH, LIFE and POWER!!!!!

What is Critical Reading?

- Also known as active reading
- Paying attention to what you are reading
- Understanding the main idea (thesis statement)
- Discovering the author's purpose
- Identifying conclusions
- Maintain interest in the material

Reading and the Brain-Mind Connection

The brain-mind connection works very hard to translate the content of language. Regardless of whether the container is a Sanskrit tablet or a microchip, the energy needed to process the content is enormous.

The ability of the human mind to translate language into symbolic representation has evolved over thousands of years.

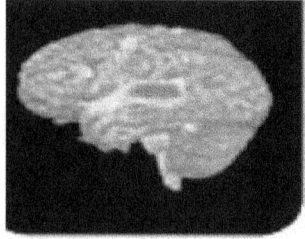
Hearing Words

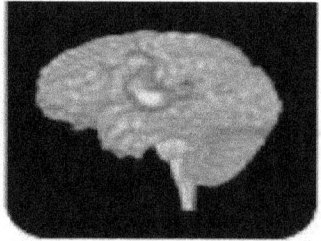
Speaking Words

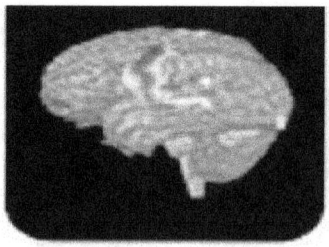
Seeing Words

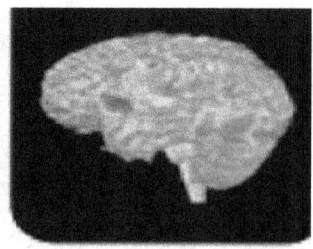
Thinking about Words

Affirm * Confirm * Claim Your Life!

Today the working memory of the mind has reached a level of sophistication that allows it to orchestrate the interaction of critical thinking, critical reading, and critical writing.

When you read, your brain "engages you in a variety of mental or cognitive processes: attention, memory, visual, auditory, and linguistic processes" (Wolf, 2009, p. 4).

When confronted with a page of words, you begin to use your critical reading skills, by:

Planning how to read at a pace that still allows you to understand the message. Next your visual system races into action, swooping quickly across the page forwarding its gleanings about letter shapes, word forms, and common phrases to linguistic systems awaiting the information. These systems rapidly connect subtly to differentiated visual symbols with essential information about the sounds contained in words demonstrating your brain's uncanny ability to connect and integrate at rapid fire speeds what it sees and what it hears to what it knows. (Wolf, 2009, p. 225)

The effort required of the human mind to be able to work with language is significant. Reading on digital hardware instead of paper still requires deep reading, which engages and exercises the brain-mind connection in a more robust and expansive way than skimming for basic, literal meaning.

It's the difference between taking a leisurely stroll and training for a marathon.

In this case, you will be reading YOUR OWN WORDS!

The Words that fills the containers of Language will be YOUR OWN ... So when you read these words, Your Brain-Mind Connection is Activated and Increased by Your Words – Unlocking YOUR Ability to HEAL YOURSELF, Increase and Improve YOUR HEALTH, Become Imbued with LIFE and Make Manifest YOUR POWER!!!!

Your Body is Created to and already works to Heal itself. We interfere with the Healing Process by Our Thought, Eating and Exercise habits.

This is YOUR TIME to Critically WRITE and READ Your Own Story of Healing, Health, Life, Power and Greatness!!!!!

Now all YOU have to DO is WALK INTO YOUR BEAUTIFUL, POWERFUL, HEALTHY, AWESOME STORY

Affirm * Confirm * Claim Your Life!

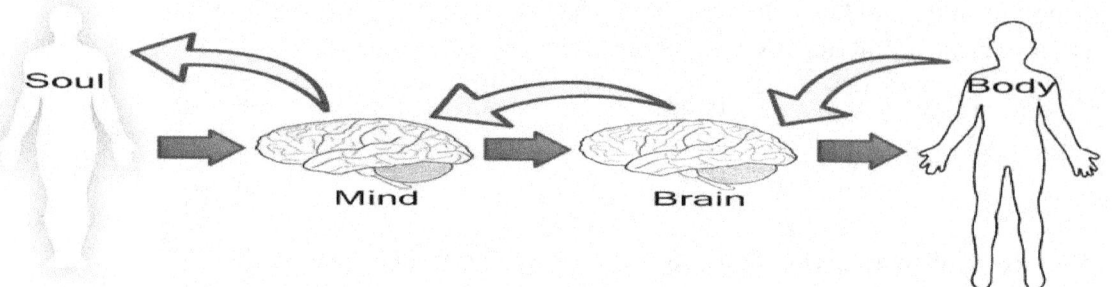

The Benefits of Deep Reading

Critical reading is deep reading. Deep reading helps you "to uncover the invisible world that resides in written words" (Wolf, 2009, p. 226). Deep reading allows you, the reader, to go beyond the information given.

Deep reading engages you in interpreting text and making rich mental connections by picking up on contextual clues and making predictions based upon signs and evidence embedded in the text.

Deep reading also involves paying attention to, rather than skipping over, the symbols, numbers, and graphs found in the written directions, plans, manuals, and blueprints, otherwise known as "visual jargon" (Rose, 2004, p. 205). Workers use critical reading with numbers on tools and gauges—in order to understand them as pressures, temperatures, progressions of processes, and so on—and on ingredient tables, spreadsheets, invoices, production quotas, shift logs, codes, and bills of lading; all this forms a significant part of "literacy in the work place" (Rose, 2004, p. 206).

With this book, you will be engaged in DEEP READING ABOUT YOURSELF!!

The text that you will be interpreting and the rich mental connections you make will create will be ABOUT YOU!!!

You will gain a Deeper Understanding of YourSelf – becoming an Expert of Yourself …. Able to Successfully make Manifest YOUR Healing, Health, Life Power and GREATNESS!!!

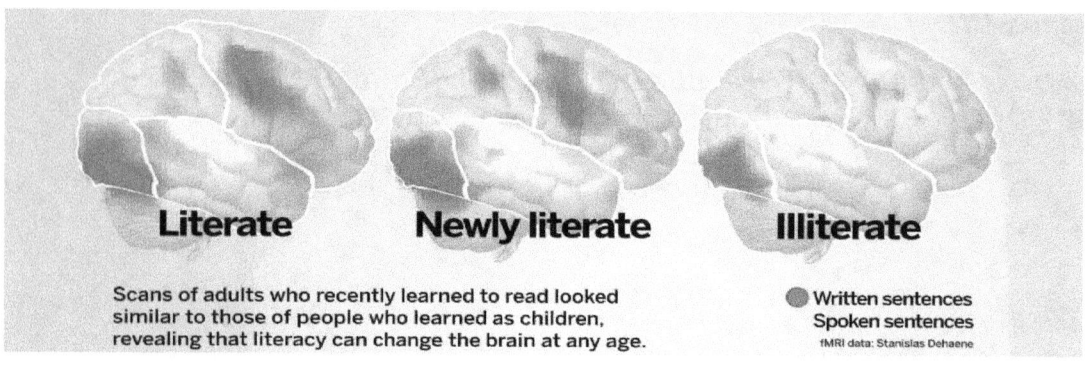

Scans of adults who recently learned to read looked similar to those of people who learned as children, revealing that literacy can change the brain at any age.

● Written sentences
● Spoken sentences
fMRI data: Stanislas Dehaene

The ultimate brain workout

Different physical exercises can bring specific mental gains, from improving memory to dealing with cravings or reducing stress

LIFTING WEIGHTS
Prefrontal cortex
complex thinking,
reasoning, multitasking,
problem-solving

YOGA
Frontal lobe
Insula
integrates thoughts
and emotions

Amygdala
fear and anxiety

HIGH-INTENSITY INTERVALS
Hypothalamus
appetite regulation,
cravings and addiction

SPORTS DRILLS
Prefrontal cortex
Basal ganglia
attention, switching
between tasks, inhibition

Parietal lobe
visual-spacial
processing

Cerebellum
attention

AEROBIC EXERCISE
Hippocampus
memory

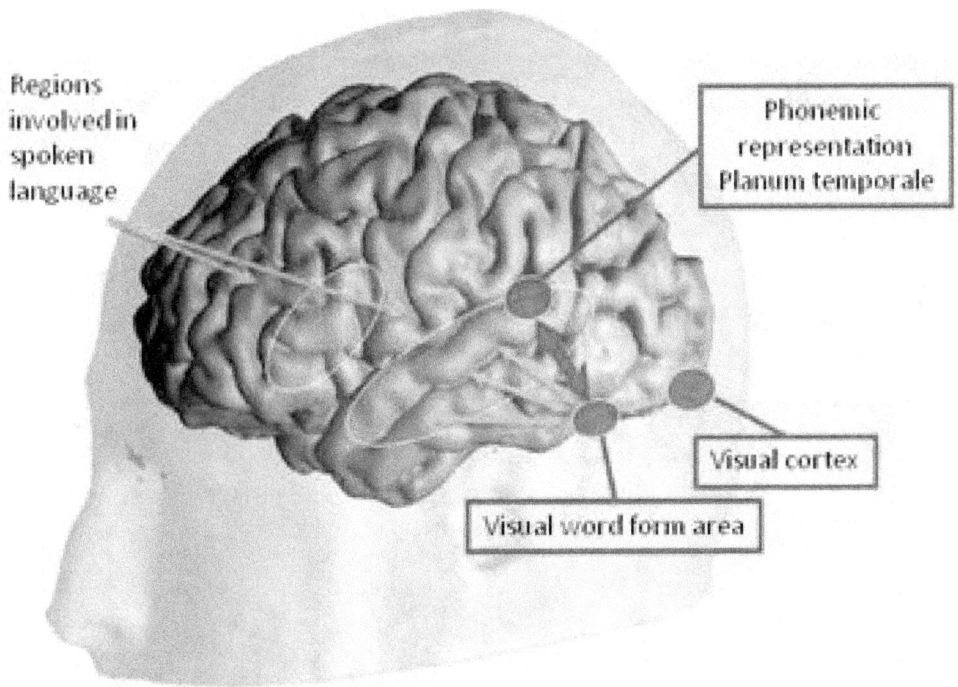

Regions involved in spoken language

Phonemic representation
Planum temporale

Visual cortex

Visual word form area

*Affirm * Confirm * Claim Your Life!*

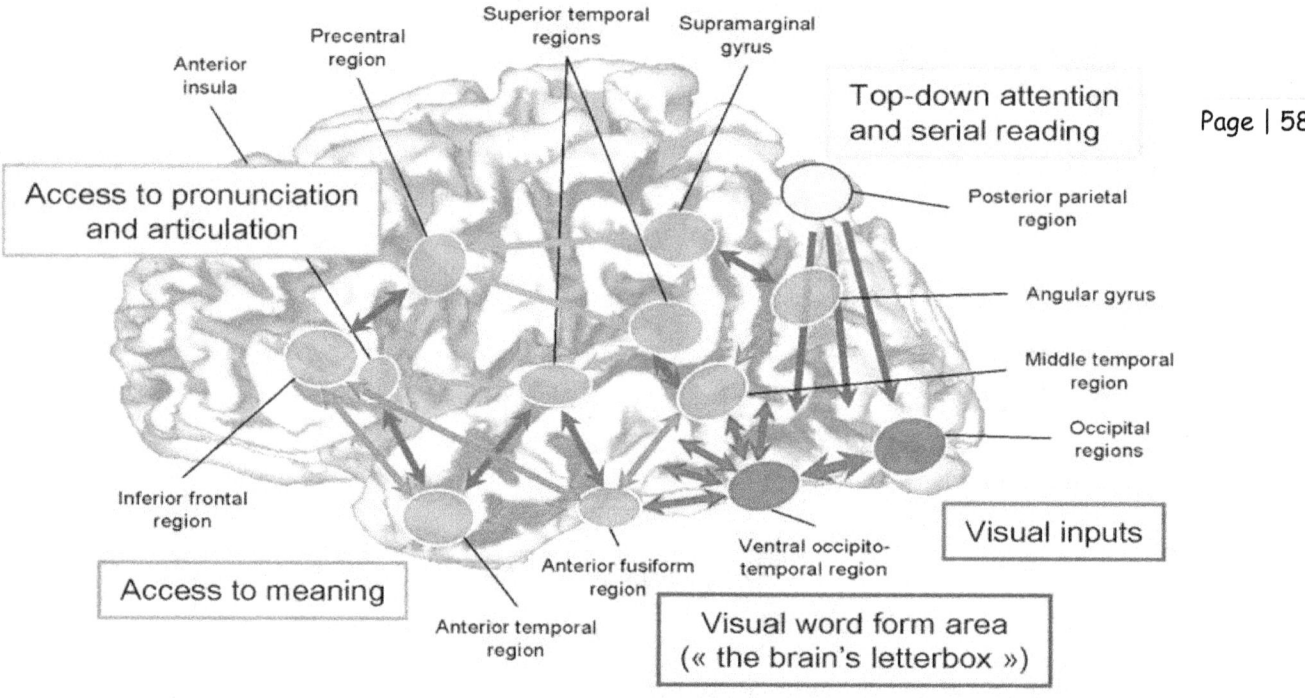

A modern vision of the cortical networks for reading

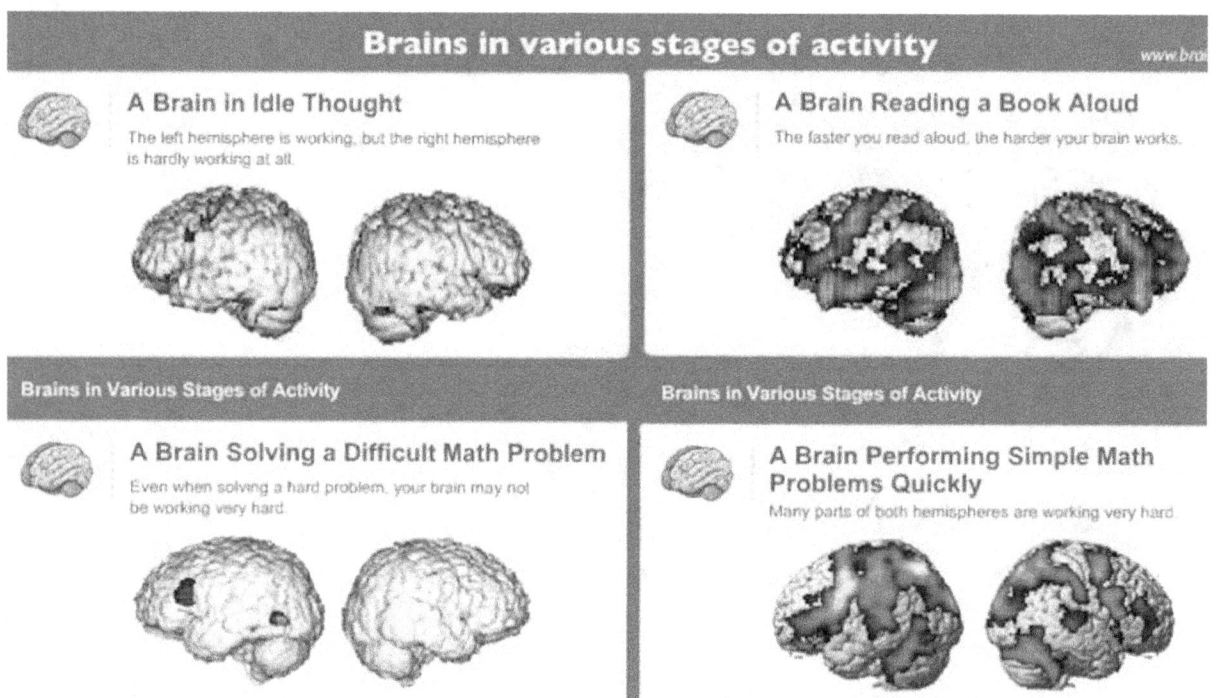

*Affirm * Confirm * Claim Your Life!*

_____'s Self-Assessment

Why Complete a Self-Assessment?

Completing a self-assessment takes a snapshot of your life, where you are at right now, and helps you to determine what's important to you at this moment.

Directions

In each space, reflect on what's going on in your life in each of these parts of your life. Write a few words or phrases that capture what it is happening or needs to change.

Measuring Progress

In a few months (and without looking at previous self-assessments) complete another one to see where you are at. What changed? How are things the same or different? What do you want to work on?

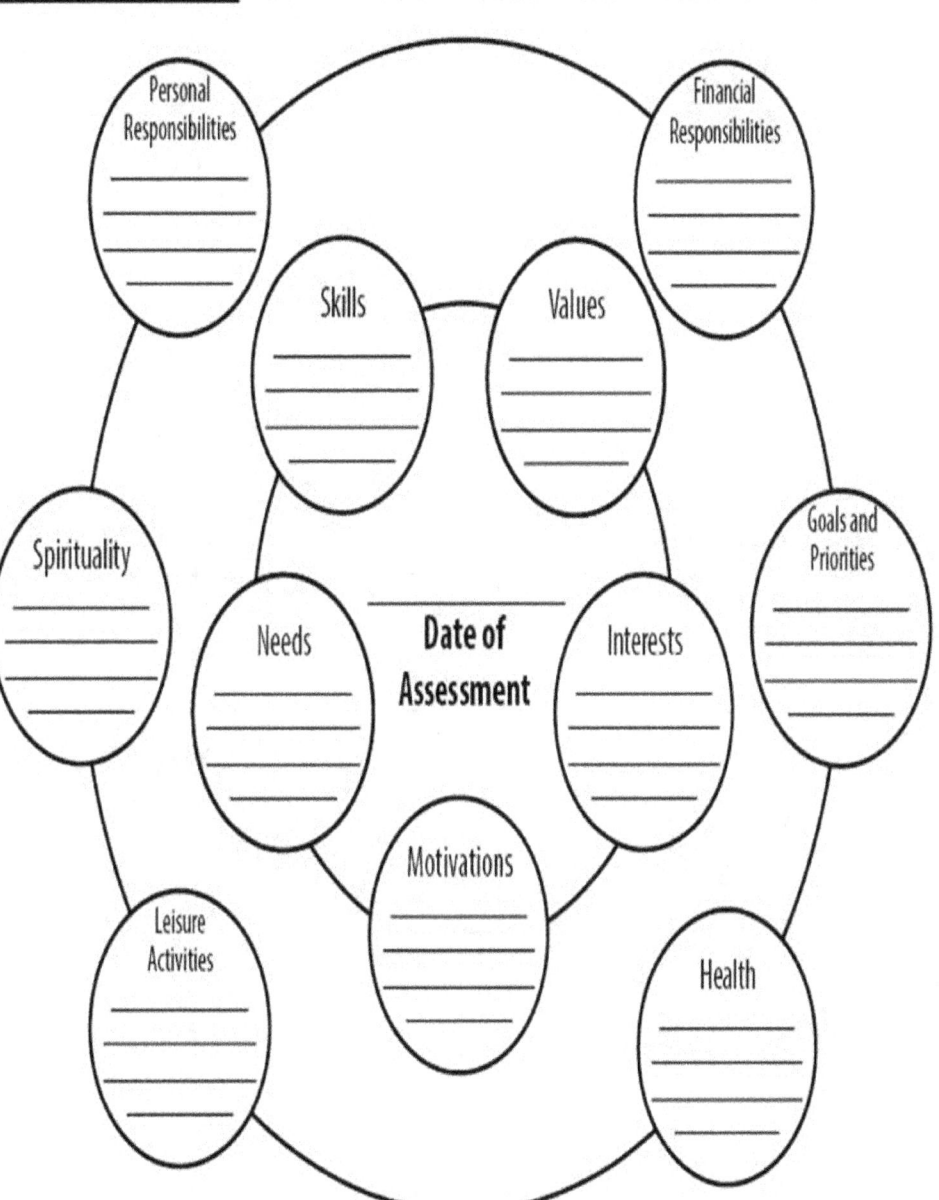

*Affirm * Confirm * Claim Your Life!*

Draw a self portrait	# WHO AM I?	
	Full Name	
	Places I have lived	Course and Section:
		Graduating Class
		Major
		Minor(s)
		Birthday
		Hobbies and extra-curricular activities
	Most memorable recent event	
An accomplishment I am proud of		Person I look up to / Pets
I have never	## Favorite — Color, Artist/Song, Sports Team, Food, TV Show, Class taken, Book, Movie	
Qualities of a good math teacher		
Something interesting about myself		

Supreme Health & Fitness!   *Knowledge Of Self Series Vol 2!*

*Affirm * Confirm * Claim Your Life!*

Self-Awareness Test

To determine your own level of awareness, read the items below and place a check mark (Y) in the blank which you think describes how often you feel this way.

	Always	Frequently	Sometimes	Rarely	Never
I'm eager to learn					
I am excited about working.					
I'm willing to listen with an open mind.					
I constantly have new ideas.					
I like taking direction from people who know something I don't.					
I try to look at the world through the eyes of the other person.					
I believe each person is unique.					

Affirm * Confirm * Claim Your Life!

My Strengths and Qualities

Things I am good at:
1 _____
2 _____
3 _____

Compliments I have received:
1 _____
2 _____
3 _____

What I like about my appearance:
1 _____
2 _____
3 _____

Challenges I have overcome:
1 _____
2 _____
3 _____

I've helped others by:
1 _____
2 _____
3 _____

Things that make me unique:
1 _____
2 _____
3 _____

What I value the most:
1 _____
2 _____
3 _____

Times I've made others happy:
1 _____
2 _____
3 _____

*Affirm * Confirm * Claim Your Life!*

Life Satisfaction

How satisfied are you with your life?

Give a SCORE, out of 10, for how SATISFIED you are with your life overall. (10 is very satisfied)

1   2   3   4   5   6   7   8   9   10

Give a SCORE for how much FUN you are having in life. (10 means lots of fun!)

1   2   3   4   5   6   7   8   9   10

Is there an area of your life that you could make more exciting? Briefly describe.

4. What areas of your life do you want to improve? I want to:
   - ☐ Improve my relationship.
   - ☐ Heal my heart.
   - ☐ Understand my life purpose.
   - ☐ Learn to be more efficient with time management
   - ☐ Feel more confident.
   - ☐ Change, or move forwards, my career.
   - ☐ Achieve my goals.
   - ☐ Be happier in life.
   - ☐ Live my life with ease and flow, rather than stress and frustration.
   - ☐ Feel more at peace.
   - ☐ To Learn to trust myself more/Be my Authentic Self.
   - ☐ Other _____

5. I am ready to take ACTION and make changes in my environment, habits and life.

   Maybe / Yes / No   (please circle)

*Affirm * Confirm * Claim Your Life!*

Self-Esteem Check-Up

Directions: Rate from 0 to 10 how much you believe each statement. '0' means you do not believe it at all and '10' means you completely believe it.

Statement	Rating
1. I believe in myself	_____
2. I am just as valuable as other people	_____
3. I would rather be me than someone else	_____
4. I am proud of my accomplishments	_____
5. I feel good when I get compliments	_____
6. I can handle criticism	_____
7. I am good at solving problems	_____
8. I love trying new things	_____
9. I respect myself	_____
10. I like the way I look	_____
11. I love myself even when others reject me	_____
12. I know my positive qualities	_____
13. I focus on my successes and not my failures	_____
14. I'm not afraid to make mistakes	_____
15. I am happy to be me	_____
Total Score	_____

Overall, how would you rate your self esteem on the following scale:

0_____10

I completely dislike who I am   I completely like who I am

What would need to change in order for you to move up one point on the rating scale? (i.e. For example, if you rated yourself a "6" what would need to happen for you to be at a "7"?)

_____
_____
_____
_____

Supreme Health & Fitness!   Knowledge Of Self Series Vol 2!

*Affirm * Confirm * Claim Your Life!*

Goals and Dreams

What are your goals and dreams?

What are you most passionate about?

Where can you see yourself in ten years?

*Affirm * Confirm * Claim Your Life!*

How I Feel

I feel: _____

Happy	Mad	Sad	Glad
Worried	Excited	Bored	Scared
Annoyed	Upset	Sick	Nervous

I feel this way because:

_____
_____
_____

This is what I did about it:

_____
_____
_____

Something else I could have done is:

_____
_____
_____

| Ask for help | Take deep breaths | Walk away |
| Do something else | Tell an adult | Talk to a friend |

*Affirm * Confirm * Claim Your Life!*

Self-Awareness

Please identify where you feel you are currently on the following scales. This will help you become more self-aware of your current situation.

Self Esteem

Low   1   2   3   4   5   6   7   8   9   10   High

Happiness

Depressed   1   2   3   4   5   6   7   8   9   10   Happy

Assertiveness

Timid   1   2   3   4   5   6   7   8   9   10   Assertive

Calmness

Explosive   1   2   3   4   5   6   7   8   9   10   Calm

Life Stresses

Out of Control   1   2   3   4   5   6   7   8   9   10   Controlled

Time Management

Disorganised   1   2   3   4   5   6   7   8   9   10   Organised

*Affirm * Confirm * Claim Your Life!*

DAILY DEVOTIONAL WORKSHEET

DATE: _____

SCRIPTURE VERSE THAT SPOKE TO ME

THINK QUALITY, NOT QUANTITY.

☐ BOOM. MEMORIZED IT.

WORD STUDY FROM MY SCRIPTURE VERSE

PRAYING THE SCRIPTURE

PERSONALIZE IT & TURN IT INTO A PRAYER.

DISTRACTION PARKING LOT

JOT IT DOWN & YOU'LL GET TO IT LATER.

MEDITATION

JOURNAL A THOUGHT OR TWO.

Supreme Health & Fitness!   Knowledge Of Self Series Vol 2!

Chapter Five

Understanding the Process of Self-Concept

*****

Who are you? What Is the Self?

How has your view of yourself changed over the years?

When we think about Ourselves, we have to 1st go to the root or foundation of HOW our first understanding of Ourselves are created. Unfortunately, our beginnings of the ideas of Ourselves are created from external influences.

Newborn babies have no ego boundaries, which define where an individual stops and the rest of the world begins (Chodorow, 1989).

Within the first year or two of life, as infants start to differentiate themselves from the rest of the world, the self begins to develop. Babies, then toddlers, then children devote enormous energy to understanding who they are. They actively seek to define themselves and to become competent in the identities they claim

This is the beginning of a self-concept: the realization that one is a separate entity.

*Affirm * Confirm * Claim Your Life!*

Energetic Self Perception

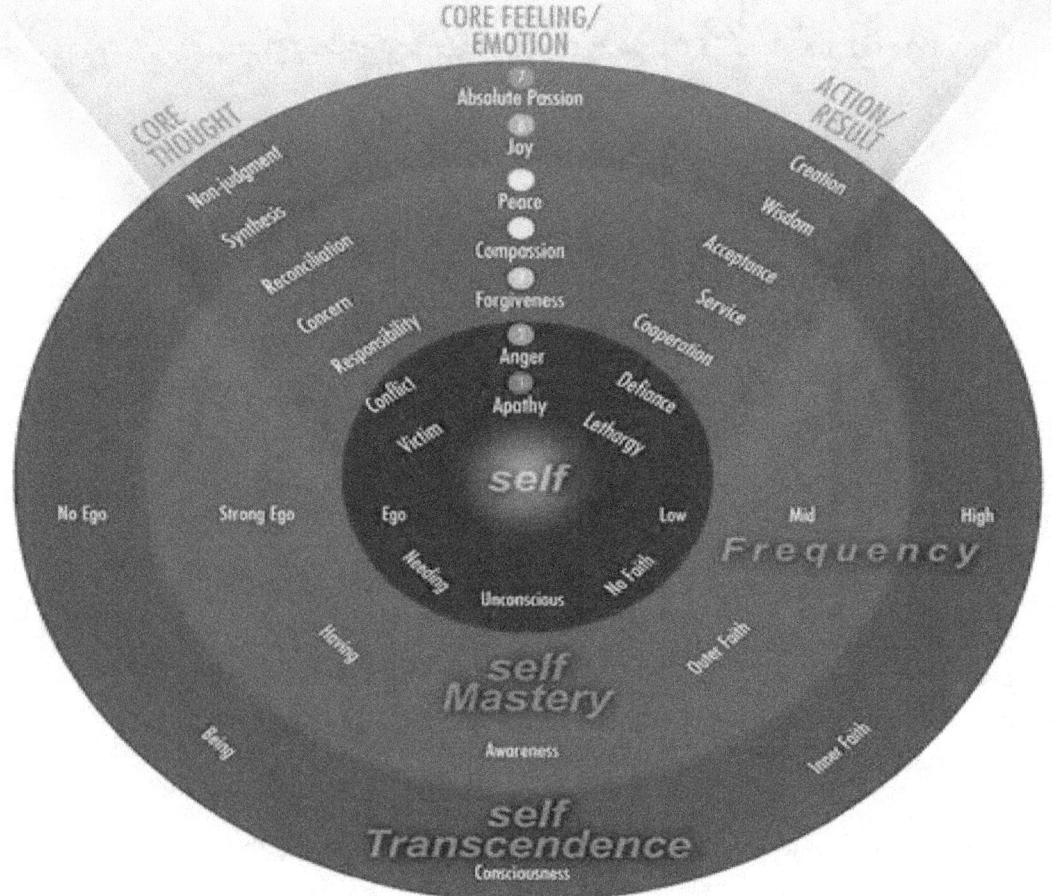

The Self arises in communication and is a multi-dimensional process of internalizing and acting from social perspectives. According to modern psychology, we develop ourselves by internalizing two kinds of perspectives that are communicated to us: the perspectives of Particular others and the perspective of the Generalized others (Mead, 1934).

Although the word Self can be construed as though it referred to a single entity, in reality the Self is made up of many dimensions.

Affirm * Confirm * Claim Your Life!

The multiple dimensions of Self are shaped and influenced by direct definitions, reflected appraisals, identity scripts, attachment styles, social comparisons, and the perspectives of the generalized other.

Once we know how the image of Ourselves is formulated, we can then examine how we, as individuals have been shaped and have the opportunity to RE-SHAPE Ourselves according to HOW we want to BE!!!!!

- **Self Concept**
  - Summarizes the beliefs a person holds about his own attributes and how he evaluates the self on these qualities
- **Ideal Self**
  - A person's conception of how he would like to be
- **Actual Self**
  - Refers to our more realistic appraisal of the qualities we do and don't have
- **Impression Management**
  - Our efforts to "manage" what others think of us; choosing products that show us off in a good light

*Affirm * Confirm * Claim Your Life!*

All About Me!

Complete these sentences about yourself. Share with others!

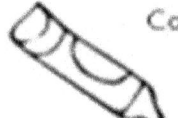

My favorite color is....	My favorite subject is....	I'm most happy when I....
The last movie I watched was....	My favorite food is	I really hate it when....
Yesterday, I....	Most people don't know that I....	If I had a million dollars....
Tomorrow, I will....	Right now, I feel very....	My favorite memory is....

Supreme Health & Fitness!   Knowledge Of Self Series Vol 2!

Affirm * Confirm * Claim Your Life!

Particular Others

The first perspectives that affects us are those of **Particular Others**. Particular others are specific people who are important in our lives.

For infants and children, the particular others include family members and caregivers. Later in life, particular others will most likely also include peers, teachers, friends, romantic partners, coworkers, and other individuals who are especially important in our lives. As babies interact with particular others in their world, they learn how others see them.

This is the beginning of a self-concept. Notice that the Self starts from outside—from how particular others view us.

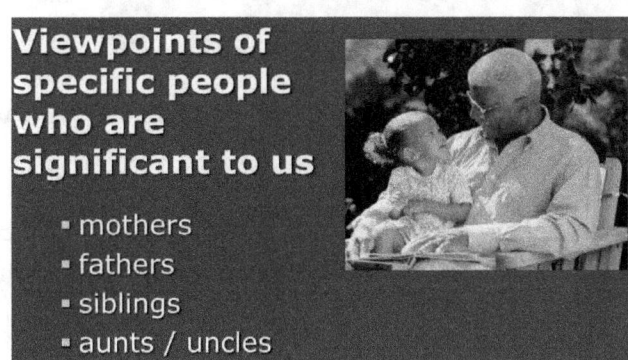

Parents and other individuals who matter to us communicate who we are and what we are worth through the concepts of direct definitions, reflected appraisals, scripts, and attachment styles.

Direct Definition

As the name implies, direct definition is communication that tells us explicitly who we are by directly labeling us and our behaviors. Family members, as well as peers, teachers, and other individuals, define us by telling us who we are or are expected to be.

Positive direct definitions enhance our self-esteem: "You're smart," "You're strong," "You're great at soccer."

Negative direct definitions can damage children's self-esteem (Brooks & Goldstein, 2001): "You're a troublemaker," "You're stupid," "You're impossible."

Negative messages can and almost always do demolish a child's sense of self-worth.

*Affirm * Confirm * Claim Your Life!*

Positive messages can and almost always do increases a child's sense of self-worth.

Communication that explicitly labels us and our behaviors

- For example, a parent might say
  - "You're my little girl."
  - "You're so responsible."
  - "You're a troublemaker."
  - "You're impossible."

Important individuals in our lives often provide us with direct definitions of our racial and ethnic identities.

In cultures with a majority race, members of minority races often make special efforts to teach children to take pride in the strength and traditions of their racial and ethnic group. Thus, the ethnic training found in many African American families stresses both positive identification with black heritage and awareness of prejudice on the part of people who are not black.

Cultures vary in how they view the self and even in when they believe social identity begins. In the United States, a person is thought to exist at least when biological birth occurs, and many Americans believe that a fetus is a human self. Yet, in some societies, the self does not start at birth—and certainly not prior to birth (Morgan, 1996).

Direct definitions can boost or impair children's self-esteem, growth, development and what type of adult they become and ultimately how they behave and achieve.

Direct definitions lead directly to Reflected Appraisals. From direct definition, children learn what others value in them, and this shapes what they come to value in themselves. They use how others described them to form HOW they describe or view themselves to themselves.

- Reflected Appraisal – perceptions of the judgements of those around us
- Judgements of significant others are especially salient.
- Social Comparison – evaluating ourselves in terms of how we compare to others
- We use reference groups as a basis of comparison.

Affirm * Confirm * Claim Your Life!

Reflected Appraisal

Reflected appraisal is our perception of another's view of us. How we think others appraise us affects how we see ourselves. This concept is similar to the ***looking-glass*** self, based on Charles Cooley's poetic comment, "Each to each a looking glass/Reflects the other that doth pass" (1961).

Others are mirrors for us—the views of ourselves that we see in them (our mirrors) shape how we perceive ourselves.

One way to think about reflected appraisals and direct definitions is to realize that others' expressed views of us can elevate or lower our self-concept. People elevate our self-concept when they admire our strengths and accomplishments and accept our weaknesses and problems without discounting us. When we're around these people, we feel more upbeat and positive about ourselves.

REFLECTED APPRAISAL

- **Others are a mirror for how we see/interpret/evaluate ourselves**
- **Mental Process**
    - "I think you believe …"
    - "I believe you believe …"
    - "I know you believe …"
- **Three Types: Uppers, Downers, Vultures**
    - Uppers
        - Admire and accept
    - Downers
        - Point out and put down
    - Vultures
        - Exploit and attach

This is what we want to accomplish with Creating and Building our own Self Definition and Self Appraisal, based on our own Love and Respect of Yourself!

We want to use our own direct definitions of ourselves to establish our own Appraisals of ourselves that will create in us the environment of Healing, Health, Power and Life.

We empower ourselves to be able to turn inward to get the Energy and Power we need to accomplish ALL our goals instea0d of having to depend on others and becoming stuck or rendering ourselves power-LESS.

Affirm * Confirm * Claim Your Life!

SELF- ESTEEM WORKSHEET

NAME_____SLS1301C – Life Career Planning

DEFINE SELF -ESTEEM:
_____
_____
_____

List 10 adjectives, positive or negative that YOU think describe you. Ex. I am creative. I am stubborn.

1._____ 6._____

2._____ 7._____

3._____ 8._____

4._____ 9._____

5._____ 10._____

List 4 of your strengths:

1._____

2._____

3._____

4._____

List 4 of your weaknesses/challenges:

1._____

2._____

3._____

4._____

Supreme Health & Fitness!   Knowledge Of Self Series Vol 2!

*Affirm * Confirm * Claim Your Life!*

How Can I Improve?

Name: _____

Date: _____

Currently I can _____
_____

I need to improve _____
_____

My goal is to _____
_____

List ways to reach your goal:
1. _____
2. _____
3. _____
4. _____
5. _____

I will achieve the goal on this date: _____

Supreme Health & Fitness!   Knowledge Of Self Series Vol 2!

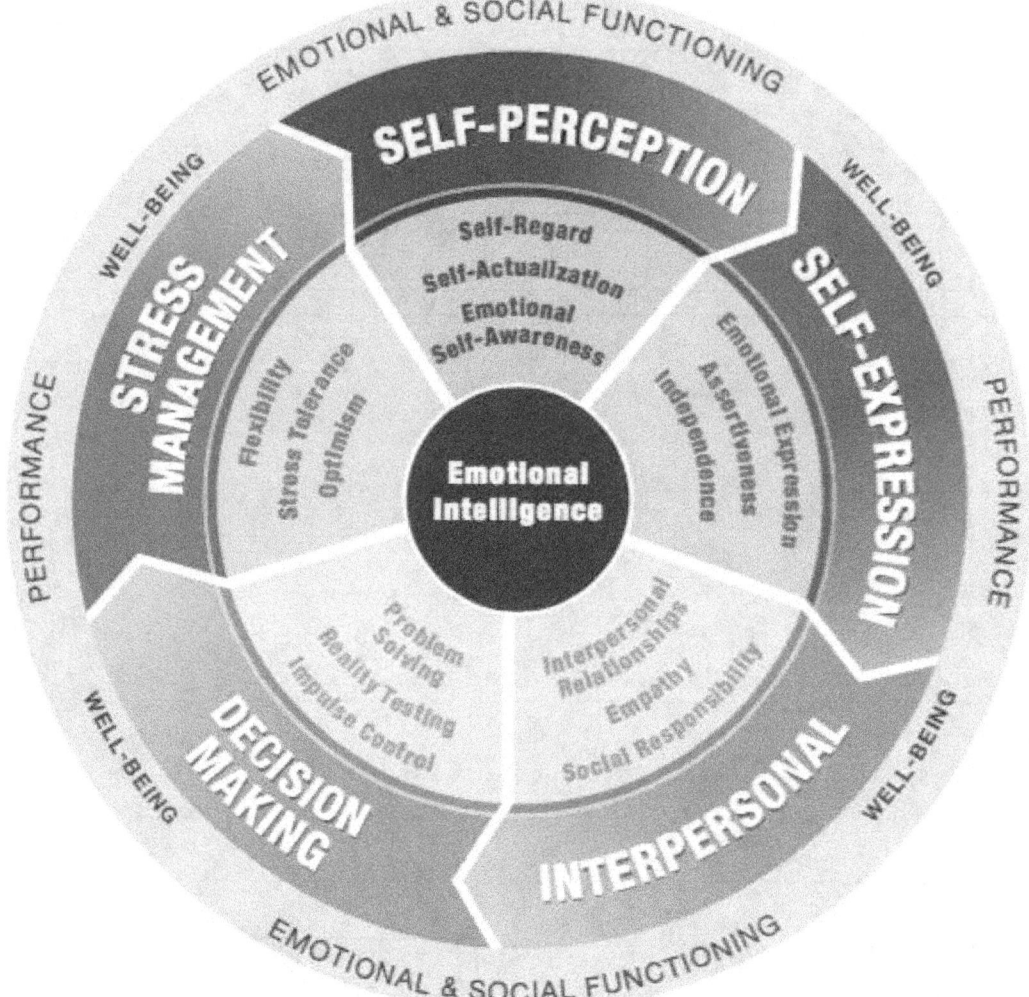

*Affirm * Confirm * Claim Your Life!*

Chapter Six

Guidelines for Improving Self-Concept

· · · · ·

So far, we have explored how we form our self-concepts as we interact with particular people and as we encounter widely held social perspectives. Now, we want to know how we can enhance our self-concepts using our own definitions and perspectives about ourselves.

Make a Firm Commitment to Personal Growth

The first principle for changing self-concept is the most difficult and the most important. You must make a firm commitment to cultivating personal growth. This isn't as easy as it might sound.

	Actual Self	Ideal Self
Private Self	How I see myself	How I would like to see myself
Public (Social) Self	How others see me	How I would like others to see me

A firm commitment involves more than saying, "I want to be more open to others." Or "I want to be more open to myself." Saying these sentences is simple and the easiest part.

You have to invest **energy** and **effort** to bring about change. From the start, realize that changing how you think of yourself is a major project.

Affirm * Confirm * Claim Your Life!

Changing how we see ourselves is a long-term process, so we can't let setbacks undermine our commitment to change. Apparently, consistency itself is comforting and we can draw the strength that we need from being consistent to the commitment of our change.

We know ourselves better than anyone else. So, if you realize in advance that you may struggle against change, you'll be prepared for the tension that accompanies personal growth. The better prepared you are the more successful you will be at controlling them.

Most failure can be found in a person knowing their struggles but not adequately preparing to encounter or overcome their overcome their known short-comings.

Gain and Use Knowledge to Support Personal Growth

Commitment alone is insufficient to bring about constructive changes in your self-concept. In addition, you need several types of knowledge. First, you need to understand how your self-concept was formed.

Second, you need information about yourself. One way to get this information is through self-disclosure, which is revealing information about ourselves that others are unlikely to discover on their own.

Self-disclosure is an important way to learn about ourselves (Greene, Derlega, & Mathews, 2006). As we reveal our hopes, fears, dreams, and feelings, we get responses from others that give us new perspectives on who we are. This enables us to understand HOW our own Mind works in a given situation.

The Johari Window

	Known to self	Not known to self
Known to others	Open	Blind
Not known to others	Hidden	Unknown

In addition, we gain insight into ourselves by seeing how we interact with others in new situations which allows us to have more or better control over our interactions so that we can get the most from them.

Affirm * Confirm * Claim Your Life!

A number of years ago, Joseph Luft and Harry Ingham (Luft, 1969) created a model of different sorts of knowledge that affect self-development.

They called the model the Johari Window, which is a combination of their first names, Joe and Harry.

Four types of information are relevant to the self:

1. **Open**, or **public**, information is known both to us and to others. Your name, height, major, and tastes in music probably are open information that you share easily with others.

2. The **blind area** contains information that others know about us but we don't know about ourselves. For example, others may see that we are insecure even though we think we've hidden that well. Others may also recognize needs or feelings that we haven't acknowledged to ourselves.

3. **Hidden information** is what we know about ourselves but choose not to reveal to most others. You might not tell many people about your vulnerabilities or about traumas in your past because you consider this private information. The unknown area is made up of information about ourselves that neither we nor others know. This consists of your untapped resources, your untried talents, and your reactions to experiences you've never had. You don't know how you will manage a crisis until you've been in one, and you can't tell what kind of parent you would be unless you've had a child.

4. The **unknown area** is made up of information about ourselves that neither we nor others know. This consists of your untapped resources, your untried talents, and your reactions to experiences you've never had. You don't know how you will manage a crisis until you've been in one, and you can't tell what kind of parent you would be unless you've had a child.

	Known to self	Not known to self
Known to Others	The areas of your life that are the so-called open book.	The blind spots – we all have them.
Not Known to Others	The things you know about yourself but will not share with others.	The things about you that no one knows, not even you.

Affirm * Confirm * Claim Your Life!

Set Goals That Are Realistic and Fair

This can be considered the most important aspect of developing your self-concept and oft-times is the catalyst between someone's failure or Success of creating their own self-concept. We set a goal for ourselves that is unobtainable which almost ensures our failure.

Efforts to change how we see ourselves work best when we set realistic and fair goals.

In a culture that emphasizes perfectionism, it's easy to be trapped into expecting more than is humanly possible.

Western society urges us to expect more and more of ourselves—more promotions and raises, more productivity, more possessions, more everything (Lacher, 2005). This type of mind-set creates an overly competitive environment that fosters an every-man-for-themselves attitude which is not conducive to Peace, Cooperation or Unity.

Peter Whybrow, who is the director of a neuroscience center, believes that Americans relentlessly seek possessions and status. He argues that the American addiction to having more of everything is futile because more is never enough; if we get more, we want even more! This is unrealistic and can only make us unhappy, because we can never achieve or have or be enough.

- **S** — **Specific:** State exactly what you want to accomplish (Who, What, Where, Why)
- **M** — **Measurable:** How will you demonstrate and evaluate the extent to which the goal has been met?
- **A** — **Achievable:** stretch and challenging goals within ability to achieve outcome. What is the action-oriented verb?
- **R** — **Relevant:** How does the goal tie into your key responsibilities? How is it aligned to objectives?
- **T** — **Time-bound:** Set 1 or more target dates, the "by when" to guide your goal to successful and timely completion (include deadlines, dates and frequency)

We should be fair to ourselves by acknowledging our strengths and virtues as well as our limitations and aspects of our- selves we want to change.

Affirm * Confirm * Claim Your Life!

Being fair to yourself also requires you to accept that you are **in process**. One across-the-board characteristic of the human self is that it is continually in process, always becoming. This implies several things.

Statement	Strongly Agree	Agree	Disagree	Strongly Disagree
1. I feel that I am a person of worth, at least on an equal plan with others.				
2. I feel that I have a number of good qualities.				
3. All in all, I am inclined to feel that I am a failure.				
4. I am able to do things as well as most other people				
5. I feel I do not have much to be proud of.				
6. I take a positive attitude toward myself.				
7. On the whole, I am satisfied with myself.				
8. I wish I could have more respect for myself				
9. I certainly feel useless at times.				
10. At times, I think I am no good at all.				

First, it means you need to accept who you are now as a starting point. You don't have to like or admire everything about yourself, but it is important to accept who you are now as a basis for going forward.

The self that you are results from all the interactions, reflected appraisals, and social comparisons you have made during your life, which was beyond our control. Once we accept this as who we are NOW, we can easily re-define ourselves according to our own definitions.

You cannot change your past, but you do not have to let it define your future.

Accepting yourself as in-process also implies that you realize you can change. Who you are is not who you will be in 5 or 10 years. Don't let yourself be hindered by defeating, self-fulfilling prophecies or the false idea that you cannot change (Rusk & Rusk, 1988).

Affirm * Confirm * Claim Your Life!

You can *easily* change if you set realistic goals, make a genuine commitment, and then work for the changes you want.

According to psychiatrist Judith Orloff (2009), we are not generous with ourselves when it comes to compassion. Orloff says that many people are not self-compassionate because they think it's the same as being self-indulgent.

We render ourselves weak and powerless by allowing negative based ideas and beliefs from others to influence how we think of ourselves and treat ourselves. Everyone has a God-Given RIGHT to be able to DEFINE themselves and to live their life according to HOW they want.

Seek Contexts That Support Personal Change

Just as it is easier to swim with the tide than against it, it is easier to change our views of ourselves when we have some support for our efforts. You can do a lot to create an environment that supports your growth by choosing contexts and people who help you realize your goals.

First, think about settings. Example - If you want to become more extroverted, put yourself in social situations rather than in libraries.

Second, think about the people whose appraisals of you will help you move toward changes you desire. You can put yourself in supportive contexts by consciously choosing to be around people who believe in you and encourage your personal growth.

It's equally important to steer clear of people who pull us down or say we can't change. In other words, people who reflect positive appraisals of us enhance our ability to improve.

One of the most crippling kinds of self-talk we can engage in is self-sabotage. This involves telling ourselves we are no good, we can't do something, there's no point in trying to change, and so forth. We may be repeating judgments others have made of us, or we may be inventing our own negative self-fulfilling prophecies. Either way, self-sabotage defeats us because it undermines belief in ourselves.

Self-sabotage is poisonous; it destroys our motivation to change and grow.

Affirm * Confirm * Claim Your Life!

We can also affirm our strengths, encourage our growth, and fortify our sense of self-worth. Positive self-talk builds motivation and belief in yourself.

It is also a useful strategy to interrupt and challenge negative messages from yourself and others.

The next time you hear yourself saying, "I can't do this" or someone else says, "You'll never change," challenge the negative message with self-talk. Say out loud to yourself, "I can do it. I will change."

Use positive self-talk to resist counterproductive communication about yourself. This creates the environment of Power IN You. Instead of wondering if you can accomplish something – YOU KNOW YOU CAN!

How true are these statements of you?	Slightly	Partly	Fairly	Mostly	Totally
I am beginning to question whether my negative picture of myself is really accurate					
I don't get so anxious or upset when I think about who I am and what I am like					
I am feeling more optimistic about what I can do in the future					
I feel more confident and relaxed generally					
I am really looking forward to making positive changes for myself					

Perceptual Process

Perceptual process are broadly classified into following major steps:

1. **Receiving stimuli :** There are five sensory organ in human organism i.e. vision, hearing, smell, touch and test stimuli receive by human body through organs.

2. **Selecting stimuli :** The body of any individual select only those stimuli which are important and this selection is governed by two set of factors viz. External and Internal.

3. **Process of organising :** The stimuli receive by any individual must be organise properly so as to assign some meaning of them.

4. **Interpreting :** After the data has been receive and organise the next step is to interpret that data.

5. **Process of checking :** After the data have been interpreted the perceiver checks whether his interpretation are proper or not.

6. **Process of reacting :** The perceiver should take some action in relation to his perception.

Affirm * Confirm * Claim Your Life!

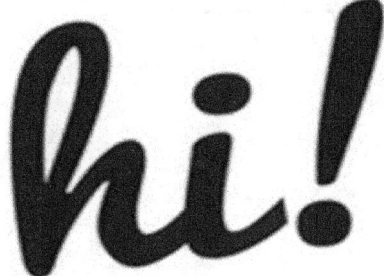

hi!
today will be...
awesome

daily goal

desired outcome

phone calls	email	media

*Affirm * Confirm * Claim Your Life!*

Self-Esteem Journal

MON.	Something I did well today...	
	Today I had fun when...	
	I felt proud when...	
TUE.	Today I accomplished...	
	I had a positive experience with...	
	Something I did for someone...	
WED.	I felt good about myself when...	
	I was proud of someone else...	
	Today was interesting because...	
THUR.	I felt proud when...	
	A positive thing I witnessed...	
	Today I accomplished...	
FRI.	Something I did well today...	
	I had a positive experience with (a person, place, or thing)...	
	I was proud of someone when...	
SAT.	Today I had fun when...	
	Something I did for someone...	
	I felt good about myself when...	
SUN.	A positive thing I witnessed...	
	Today was interesting because...	
	I felt proud when...	

Supreme Health & Fitness!   Knowledge Of Self Series Vol 2!

*Affirm * Confirm * Claim Your Life!*

SUPPORT SYSTEM

Who can I call when...

I'm feeling lonely:
_____

I need some company:
_____

I need someone to talk to:
_____

I need someone to encourage me to get out of the house and do something fun:
_____

I need someone to remind me to follow my self care plan:
_____

Other:
_____

*Affirm * Confirm * Claim Your Life!*

Positive Experiences

Write briefly about times when you displayed each of the following qualities.

Courage

Kindness

Selflessness

Love

Sacrifice

Wisdom

Happiness

Determination

*Affirm * Confirm * Claim Your Life!*

Chapter Seven

The Process of Self Perception

*****

Self-Perception is the determining factor to your how you ultimately define yourself. It is important for you to understand that your initial self-perception was given or defined to you by someone else and that you could have possibly been living your life thus far under the definitions of others. This is HOW you create the process to perceive yourself.

Perception is defined as the active process of creating meaning by selecting, organizing, and interpreting people, objects, events, situations, and other phenomena. ***Note that perception is defined as an active process.*** We want to understand the process of self-perception to use it to re-define Self and Create our own Perception based on our own Thoughts of Self.

We do not passively receive what is "out there" in the external world. Instead, we actively work to make sense of ourselves, others, and interactions. To do so, we select only certain things to notice, and then we organize and interpret what we have selectively noticed. What anything (especially ourselves) means to us depends on the aspects of it we notice and on our organization and interpretation of those aspects.

> **Perception Process**
>
> Perception is a three phase process of **selecting**, **organizing** and **interpreting information**, people, objects, events, situations and activities. You can understand interpersonal situations better if you appreciate how you and another person construct perceptions.

Thus, perception is not a simple matter of receiving external reality. Instead, we invest a lot of energy in constructing the meanings of phenomena.

*Affirm * Confirm * Claim Your Life!*

With this chapter, I want to employ the principle and science of perception to use them so that you can Actively Process your own understanding of your Self-Perception.

Perception consists of three processes: selecting, organizing, and interpreting.

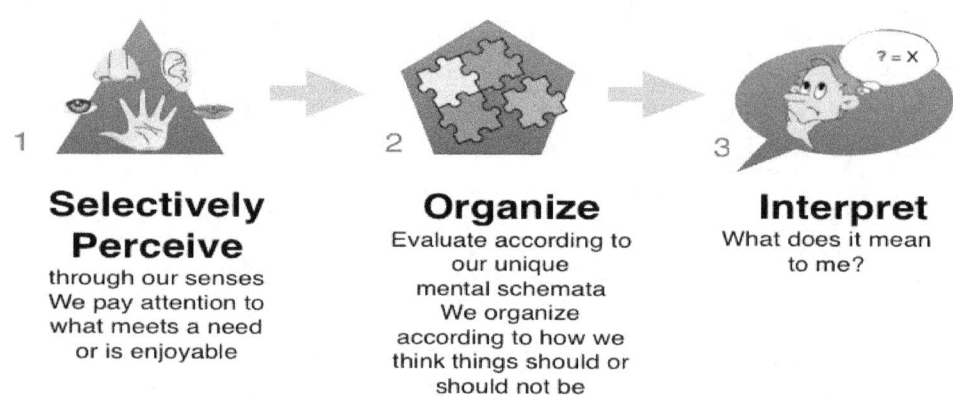

We take this science of perception and we Successfully apply it to ourselves to create or on environment of Love, Healing and Greatness Within Self!

WE scientifically Build and Create Our Own Wellness to successfully carry us into the enjoyment of Abundant LIFE!!!!

These processes are continuous, so they blend into one another. They are also interactive, so each of them affects the other two. For example, what we select to perceive in a particular situation affects how we organize and interpret the situation. At the same time, how we organize and interpret a situation affects our subsequent selections of what to perceive in the situation.

For the purposes of this book, we take the principles of HOW Perception is developed to create how we Perceive, Organize and Interpret ourselves.

Selection

Stop for a moment and notice what is going on around you right now. Is there music in the background? Is the room warm or cold, messy or neat, large or small, light or dark? Can you smell anything—food being cooked, the stale odor of last night's popcorn, traces of cologne? Can you hear muted sounds of activities outside?

Affirm * Confirm * Claim Your Life!

Now, think about what's happening inside you: Are you sleepy, hungry, comfortable? Do you have a headache or an itch anywhere? On what kind of paper is your book printed? Is the type large, small, easy to read? How do you like the size of the book, the colors used, the design of the pages?

Probably you weren't aware of most of these phenomena when you began reading the chapter. Instead, you focused on understanding the content in the book. You narrowed your attention to what you defined as important, and you were unaware of other aspects of the book and your surroundings. This is typical of how we live our lives.

This also reflects HOW we create the NEW Paradigm on View we ourselves.

We select only certain things to notice, and then we organize and interpret what we have selectively noticed.

What we select to perceive affects how we organise and interpret the situation.

How we organise and interpret a situation affects our subsequent selections of what to perceive in the situation.

We have so many definitions of ourselves – given to us be OTHERS that we MUST change to what's Important to us and NARROW your Attention on that and become un-aware of the definitions of Others!

We can't attend to everything in our environment (Internal or External), because there is far too much going on in and around us and IN us, and we don't view most of it as relevant to us in any given moment.

We select to attend to certain stimuli based on a number of factors. First, some qualities of phenomena draw attention. For instance, we notice things that STAND OUT, because they are larger, more intense, or more unusual than other phenomena. So we're more likely to hear a loud voice than a soft one and to notice bright, flashy ads on the Internet than a black-and-white message.

Change also compels attention …. The Change of YourSelf Compels YOUR ATTENTION!

Recent research shows that we can override the draw of noisy or novel stimuli (definintions from Others).

Affirm * Confirm * Claim Your Life!

We can use the prefrontal cortex, which is known as the brain's planning center, to focus our attention deliberately (Gallagher, 2009; Tierney, 2009).

We rely on self-indication when we call particular phenomena to our attention. In fact, in many ways education is a process of learning to indicate to ourselves things we hadn't seen before.

Right now, you're learning to be more conscious of the selectivity of your perceptions about yourself, so in the future you will notice this more on your own. In English courses, you learn to notice how authors craft characters and use words to create images. In science courses, you learn to attend to molecular structures and chemical reactions.

What we select to notice is also influenced by who we are and what is going on within us. Our motives and needs affect what we see and don't see. If you have recently ended a romantic relationship, you're more likely to notice attractive people at a party than if you are committed to someone.

Motives also explain the oasis phenomenon, in which thirsty people stranded in the desert see water although none really exists. In a series of experiments, researchers showed that people perceive objects they desire (water when thirsty or money) as closer than objects they do not desire (Balcetis & Dunning, in press).

Cultures also influence what we select to perceive. Assertiveness and competitiveness are encouraged and considered good in the United States, so we don't find it odd when people compete and try to surpass one another.

By contrast, because some traditional Asian cultures emphasize group loyalty, cooperation, and face saving, competitiveness is noticed and judged negatively (Gudykunst & Lee, 2002).

Organization

Once we have selected what to notice, we must make sense of it. We organize what we have noticed and attribute meaning to it.

A useful theory for explaining how we organize experience is constructivism, which states that we organize and interpret experience by applying cognitive structures called schemata

Affirm * Confirm * Claim Your Life!

We rely on four schemata to make sense of interpersonal phenomena: prototypes, personal constructs, stereotypes, and scripts (Kelly, 1955; Hewes, 1995).

> Once we selected what to notice, we must make sense of it.
> Organize in meaningful ways.
> Constructivism; we organize and interpret experience by applying cognitive structures called schemata.

Prototypes   A prototype defines the clearest or most representative examples of some category (Fehr, 1993). For example, you probably have prototypes for categories such as teachers, supervisors, friends, and coworkers. Each of these categories is exemplified by a person who is the ideal; that's the prototype.

> Prototypes; most representative example of a category. Defines categories by identifying ideal cases.
> Ideal models for friendship, family, business group, or relationship.
> Personal Construct; bipolar, mental yardstick we use to measure people and situation.
> Intelligent – unintelligent, kind – unkind.

Personal Constructs   A personal construct is a "mental yardstick" we use to measure a person or situation along a bipolar dimension of judgment (Kelly, 1955). Examples of personal constructs are intelligent–not intelligent, kind–not kind, responsible–not responsible, assertive–not assertive, and attractive–not attractive.

We rely on personal constructs to size up people and other phenomena. How intelligent, kind, responsible, and attractive is this person? Whereas prototypes help us decide into which broad category a phenomenon fits, personal constructs let us make more detailed assessments of particular qualities of people and other phenomena.

*Affirm * Confirm * Claim Your Life!*

The personal constructs we rely on shape our perceptions because we define things only in the terms of the constructs we use. Notice that we structure what we perceive and what it means by the constructs we choose to use. Thus, we may not notice qualities of people that aren't covered by the constructs we apply.

Stereotypes   A stereotype is a predictive generalization applied to a person or situation. Based on the category in which we place someone or something and how that person or thing measures up against the personal constructs we apply, we predict what he, she, or it will do. Stereotypes don't necessarily reflect actual similarities between people.

> Stereotype; predictive generalization about individuals and situations based on the category into which we place them.
> May be accurate or inaccurate.
> Scripts; guide to action in particular situation.
> A sequence of activities that define what we and others are expected to do in specific situation.
> Daily activities – dating, talking to professors, dealing with clerks, interacting with co-workers

Instead, stereotypes are based on our perceptions of similarities between people or on social perspectives that we've internalized. We may perceive similarities that others don't, and we may fail to perceive ways in which a phenomenon is different from the group on which a stereotype is based.

Research shows that a majority of Americans of all races have racial stereotypes that lead them to have an unconscious preference for white people over black people. You read that correctly—black people as well as people of other races favor white people (Nosek & Hansen, 2008).

Cultural critic Raina Kelley, who is African American, recounts a time when she assumed a black man at a party might be a criminal. She says "Being black doesn't get me a pass on unconscious negative feelings about African Americans" (2009, p. 28).

Scripts   The final cognitive schema we use to organize perceptions is the script. A script is a guide to action. Scripts consist of sequences of activities that are expected of us and others in particular situations.

Affirm * Confirm * Claim Your Life!

They are based on our experiences and observations of interaction in various contexts. Many of our daily activities are governed by scripts, although we're typically not aware of them. We have a script for greeting casual acquaintances on campus ("Hey, what's up?" "Not much"). You also have scripts for managing conflict, talking with professors, dealing with clerks, and interacting with coworkers on the job.

Scripts are useful in guiding us through many of our interactions. However, they are not always accurate or constructive, so we shouldn't accept them uncritically.

Similarly, if you grew up in a community that treated people of certain races negatively, you may want to assess that script critically before using it to direct your own activities.

The four cognitive schemata we have discussed interact with one another. Prototypes, personal constructs, stereotypes, and scripts are cognitive schemata that we use to organize our perceptions of people and phenomena. These cognitive schemata reflect the perspectives of particular others and the generalized other. As we interact with people, we internalize our culture's ways of classifying, measuring, and predicting phenomena and its norms for acting in various situations.

> Organize our thinking about people and situation.
> Make sense of what we notice and figure out how to act.
> Social perspectives and cultural views.

We are born into and live the 1ˢᵗ Stage of our lives under a pre-determined Script that is written by Others. The unfortunate thing is that many people NEVER get the opportunity to develop or live according to their own Script.

With this book, You will create Your Own Script of Healing, Your Own Script Of Life, Your Own Script of Power and Your Own Script of GREATNESS!!!

Influences on Perception

<u>Physiology</u>   One reason perceptions vary among people is that we differ in our sensory abilities and physiologies.

Our physiological states also influence perception. If you are tired or stressed, you're likely to perceive things more negatively than you normally would.

For instance, a playful insult from a coworker might anger you if you were feeling down but wouldn't bother you if you were feeling good.

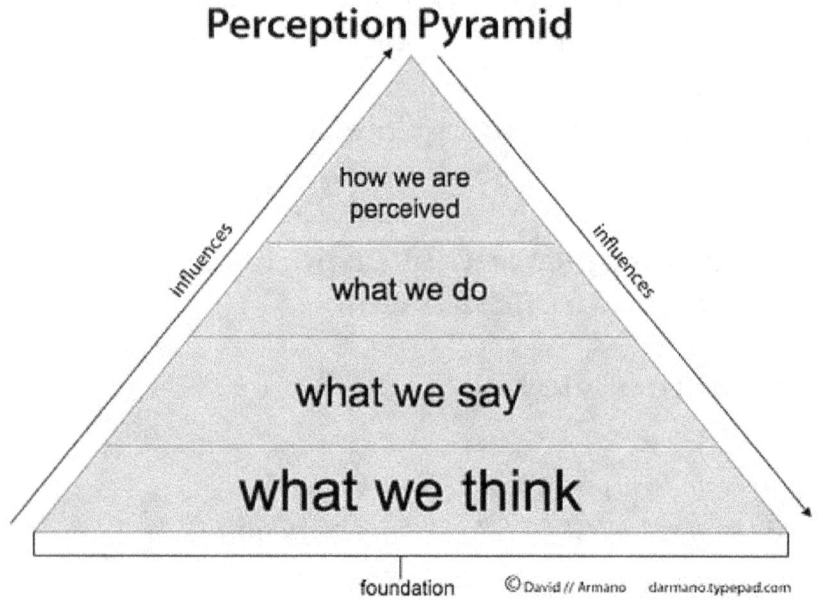

Each of us has our own bio-rhythm, which influences the times of day when we tend to be alert or fuzzy. I'm a morning person, so that's when I prefer to teach classes and write.

I am less alert and less creative later in the day. Thus, I perceive things in the morning that I simply don't notice when my energy level declines.

*Affirm * Confirm * Claim Your Life!*

- **Hunger**
  - People often get grumpy when they're hungry
  - Several biological changes occur in the body
- **Biological Cycles**
  - Your body changes constantly throughout your daily cycle
  - Change influences your perception positively and negatively
- **Psychological Challenges**
  - Mental illness and disorder can dramatically change the way one interacts with and perceives the world

Expectations   The impact of expectations on perception explains the self-fulfilling prophecy. A child who is told she is unlovable may notice rejecting, but not affirming, communication from others. An employee who is told he has leadership potential is likely to notice all his professional successes and strengths, and to be less aware of his shortcomings.

- **Expectations**
  - Preconceptions about what we are suppose to perceive may influence perception by causing us to delete, insert or modify what we see

Expectations influence perceptions in a range of communication situations. If you are told that a newly hired person is a "real team player," you're likely to notice the new employee's cooperative behaviors and be less aware of her competitive behaviors.

Age   Age is another factor that influences our perceptions. Compared with a person of 20, a 60-year-old has a more complex fund of experiences to draw on in perceiving situations and people. Age also influences our perceptions of time. My 7-year-old nephew perceives a year as much longer than I do.

A year is a full seventh of his life but less than a fiftieth of mine; a year really is longer in his life than mine.

As we grow older and have more experiences, our perspective on many things changes.

Age
- Older people view the world differently because they have a greater scope of experiences

Health and Fatigue
- How do you experience the world:
  - When you are tired?
  - When you are sick?
  - When you're hungry?
  - When you feel less sociable?

Affirm * Confirm * Claim Your Life!

Medical conditions are another physiological influence on perceptions. If you've ever taken drugs that affected your thinking, you know how dramatically they can alter perceptions. People may become severely depressed, paranoid, or uncharacteristically happy under the influence of hormones or drugs.

Changes in our bodies caused by medical conditions may also affect what we selectively perceive. I have a back disorder that periodically limits my mobility. When my back is out of order, I am far more aware of stairs, uneven ground, and any activities

Culture A culture is the totality of beliefs, values, understandings, practices, and ways of interpreting experience that are shared by a number of people.

- Research has supported the conclusion that people who live in cultures without long, parallel figures are less likely to report the top line being the longer figure.

- These results strongly support the argument that a person's experiences affect their perceptions.

Culture forms the patterns of our lives and guides how we think, feel, and communicate. The influence of culture is so pervasive that it's hard to realize how powerfully it shapes our perceptions.

Social Location In recent years, scholars have realized that we are affected not only by the culture as a whole but by particular social locations, which are defined by the social groups to which we belong (Hallstein, 2000; Haraway, 1988; Harding, 1991; Wood, 2005). A standpoint is a point of view shaped by political awareness of the social location of a group—the material, social, and symbolic conditions common for members of a social group. People who belong to powerful, high-status social groups have a vested interest in preserving the system that gives them privileges; thus, they are unlikely to perceive its flaws and inequities.

Conversely, those who belong to less-privileged groups are able to see inequities and discrimination (Collins, 1998; Harding, 1991).

Racial–ethnic groups are also social locations that shape our perceptions. Stan Gaines (1995), who studies minority groups in the United States, reports that African Americans and Latinos and Latinas tend to perceive family and extended community as more central to their identities than most European Americans do.

> - **Gender Roles**
>   - Socially instructed ways men and women should act
>   - Violations to these rules is seen as unusual and undesirable
> - **Occupational Roles**
>   - Depends on level of experience
>   - Can change instantly when new people are added to the group
>   - Philip Zimbardo conducted the an experiment that popularized the theory of occupational roles
>   - Prisoners and Guards (pg. 101-102)

Roles   Our perceptions also are shaped by roles. Both the training we receive to fulfill a role and the actual demands of the role affect what we notice and how we interpret and evaluate the role.

> **Gender role:** *the behaviors expected of people related to their identity as men and women*
>
> **Gender identity:** *one's sense of whether one is male and female, including a sense of what it means to be that gender*
>
> **Does culture define which behaviors fill a gender role? Or do the roles affect culture?**
>
> Gender roles and culture: Expectations may vary
>
> - In North American societies, men have been providers, women were caretakers
> - In some societies, men and women share more in child rearing and accumulating resources
>
> - Gender roles have simplified, yet constrained, choices for men and women.
> - In the past century, women have been gaining more options for participation in workplaces and politics.

Cognitive Abilities

In addition to physiological, cultural, and social influences, perception is also shaped by cognitive abilities. How elaborately we think about situations and people, and our personal knowledge of others, affect how we select, organize, and interpret experiences.

Cognitive Abilities—how we think about situations and people, and our personal knowledge of others

- **Cognitive complexity** *is the number of constructs, how abstract they are, and how they interact.*
- **Person-centeredness** *is the ability to perceive another as a unique individual apart from social roles and group generalizations.*

Cognitive Complexity People differ in the number and type of cognitive schemata they use to perceive, organize, and interpret people and situations.

Cognitive complexity refers to the number of personal constructs used (remember, these are bipolar dimensions of judgment), how abstract they are, and how elaborately they interact to shape perceptions.

Self

A final influence on our perceptions is ourselves. People with secure attachment styles assume that they are lovable and that others are trustworthy. Thus, they tend to perceive others and relationships in positive ways. In contrast, people with fearful attachment styles perceive themselves as unlovable and others as not loving. Consequently, they may perceive relationships as dangerous and potentially harmful.

Self—What we selectively perceive and how we organize and interpret phenomena are shaped by many aspects of our selves.
- *Attachment style*
- *Implicit personality theory is unspoken and sometimes unconscious assumptions about how various qualities fit together in human personality.*

The dismissive attachment style inclines people to perceive themselves positively, others negatively, and close relationships as undesirable.

The concept of the implicit personality theory helps explain how *the self* has influence on our interpersonal perceptions. An implicit personality theory is a collection of unspoken and sometimes unconscious assumptions about how various qualities fit together in human personalities.

*Affirm * Confirm * Claim Your Life!*

The Power of Self-Compassion

How often are we actually grateful to ourselves?
When we take note of our positive qualities, and celebrate our lives and ourselves, we become not only happier, but more successful. It helps to see yourself as you really are. Even if you see real weakness, addressing them from a place of self-compassion will help you thrive. Here are some tips for how to make self-compassion a habit:

Notice Your Self-Talk

In times of failure or challenge, noticing your self-talk can help you replace it with self-compassion. Instead of saying things like "I'm such an idiot!" you might say "I had a moment of absentmindedness and that's okay."

Write Yourself a Letter

When your emotions are overhwhelming, write a letter to yourself as if you were writing to a friend. It might feel strange at first, but your comforting words will help to normalize the situation rather than blow it out of proportion.

Develop a Self-Compassion Phrase

Use a mantra or a phrase that you can turn to in challenging situations, so you can deal with them calmly and with grace. Dr. Kristin Neff, a self-compassion researcher, uses the mantra "This is a moment of suffering. Suffering is part of life. May I be kind to myself in this moment; may I give myself the compassion I need."

Make a Daily Gratitude List

Write down 5 things you feel grateful for every day, or are proud of having accomplished. This may sound overly simplistic, but this extremely short exercise can produce powerful and long-lasting results.

*Affirm * Confirm * Claim Your Life!*

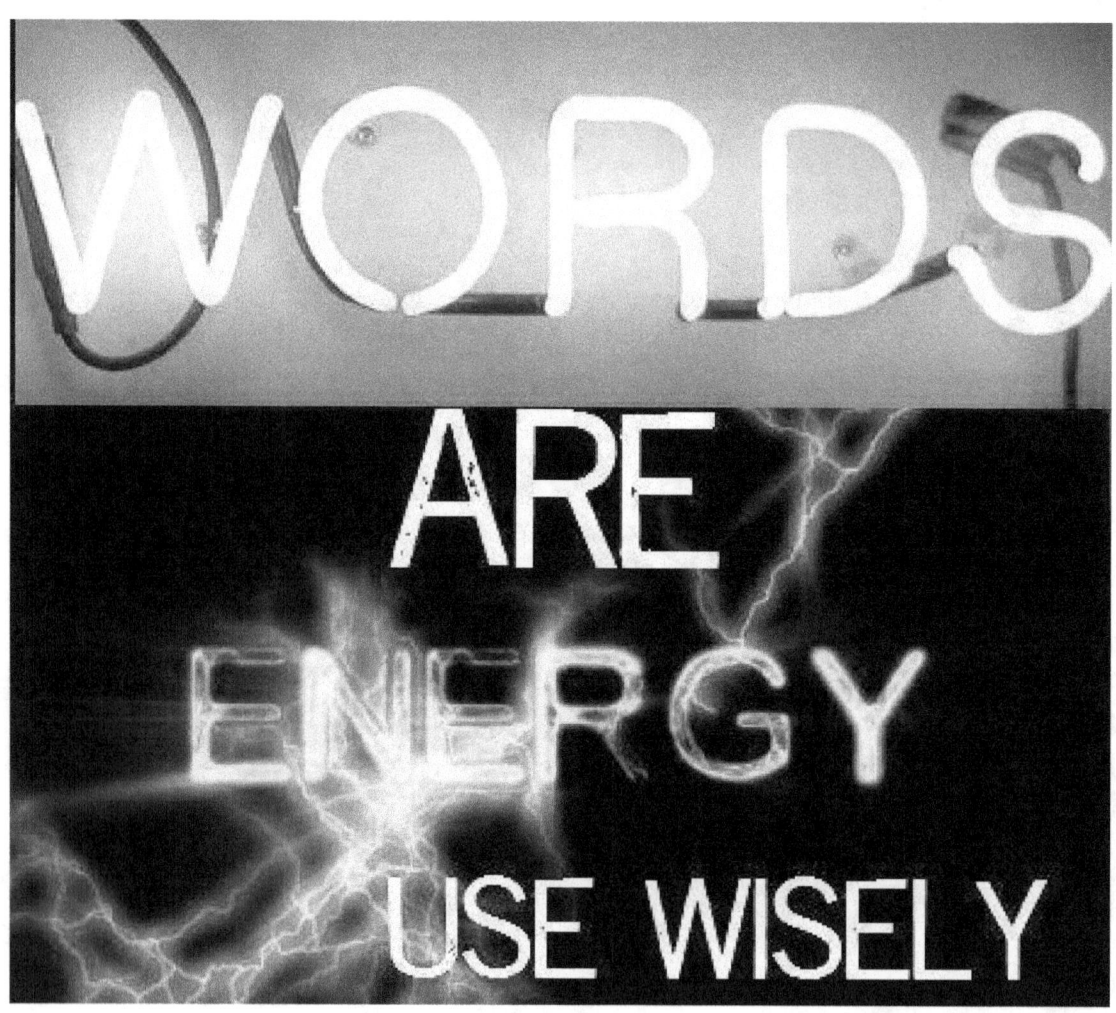

Affirm * Confirm * Claim Your Life!

Self Care Checklist

- ☐ Overspend, overeat, and overindulge
- ☐ Expect others to read your mind and meet your needs
- ☐ Withhold success from yourself
- ☐ Ignore your deepest desires but seek to fulfill the desires of others
- ☐ Ignore your real emotions and put on a "happy" face
- ☐ Push yourself beyond reasonable limits
- ☐ Allow others to emotionally, physically, or sexually abuse you
- ☐ Deflect compliments
- ☐ Say yes because you can't say no
- ☐ Avoid time alone
- ☐ Over-exhaust yourself because of your need to feel important, needed, or worthy
- ☐ Fear emotional intimacy
- ☐ Try to do it all yourself, never asking for help
- ☐ Try to appear perfect

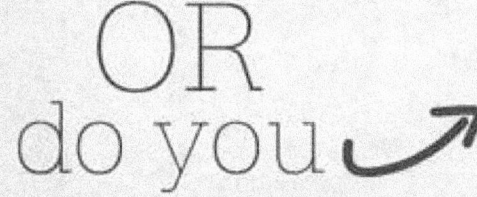

- ☐ Take time for yourself
- ☐ Allow yourself to make mistakes and to be open about your weaknesses
- ☐ Ask from your needs to be met from a place of vulnerability
- ☐ Spend time with friends
- ☐ Rest
- ☐ Play
- ☐ Exercise
- ☐ Eat well
- ☐ Spend money wisely
- ☐ Pursue your dreams
- ☐ Share honestly with others
- ☐ Enjoy and make time to enjoy and be intimate with those you love
- ☐ Forgive
- ☐ Allow others to be disappointed in you
- ☐ Appropriately express emotions, including anger and sadness
- ☐ Tell others what they mean to you
- ☐ Be present for your children
- ☐ Receive love from others
- ☐ Say yes and no
- ☐ Create a powerful support system for yourself
- ☐ Celebrate accomplishments big and small

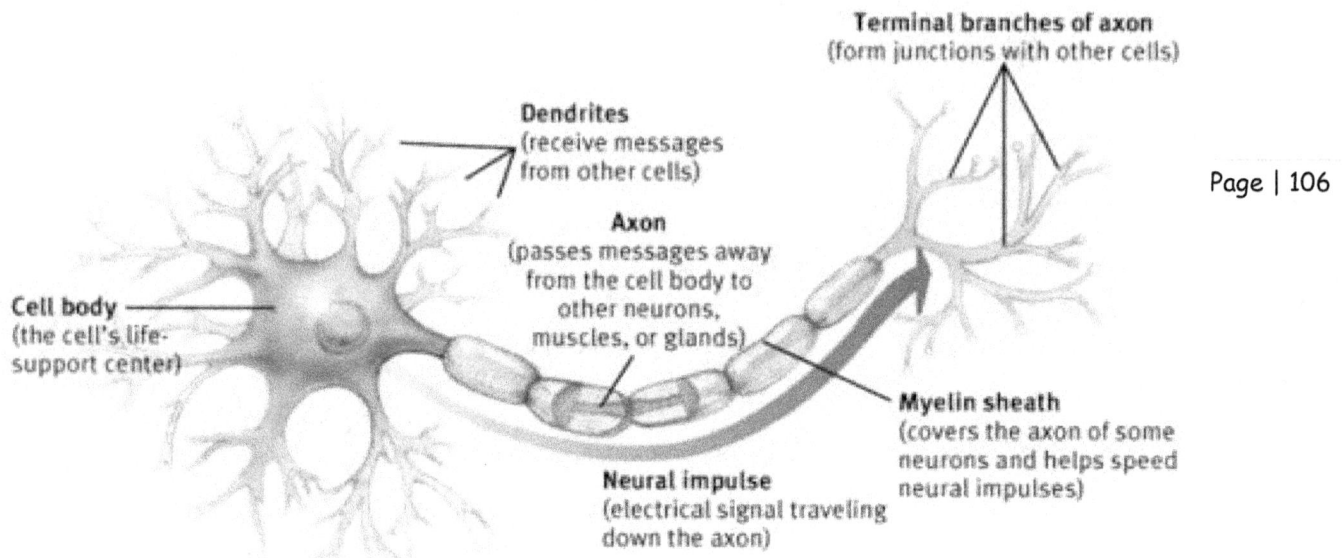

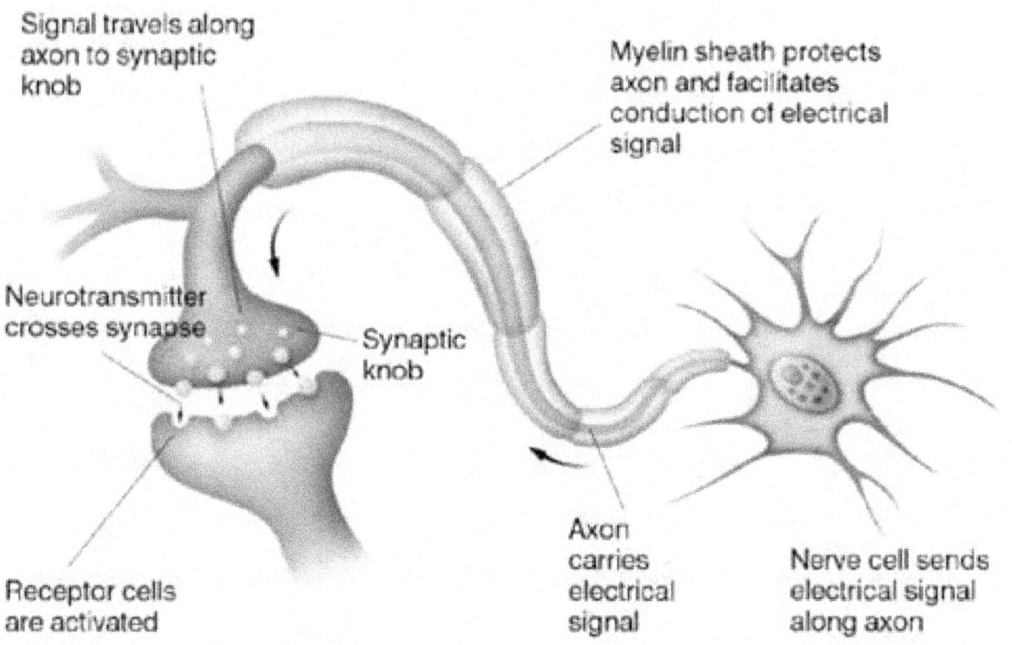

*Affirm * Confirm * Claim Your Life!*

Test Your Emotional Intelligence

This is a list of situations each followed by five possible responses (ALWAYS, USUALLY, SOMETIMES, RARELY AND NEVER).

Read each sentence carefully and out of the five possible responses, choose the one which seems to you to be the most appropriate response for a particular situation.

Always: A/ Usually: U/ Sometimes: S/ Rarely: R/ Never: N.

S.No.		A	U	S	R	N
1-	I extend help to anyone who is in need without expecting any return.					
2-	I am very sensitive and respective to the feelings of others.					
3-	I do not allow my emotions to spell to spoil my relations with others. I am always in control of my emotions.					
4-	If someone harms me in any way. I do not forget it easily; I am on a lookout to retaliate in the same coin.					
5-	I never have problem adjusting with any kind of person.					
6-	I feel guilty for any wrong that I may have done in the past.					
7-	I try to share others grief or turmoil, I am sympathetic and caring when someone is in pain.					
8-	Between the two, I get more happiness and peace of mind in giving rather than taking.					
9-	I solve a problem as soon as I confront it, and it keeps me free from worries.					
10-	I look at my problem with an open mind. I never allow my feelings and emotions to highjack my decisions and actions.					
11-	My feelings are one with the suffering person. I try to spend time with that person and share his grief and sorrow.					

Affirm * Confirm * Claim Your Life!

12-	Certain situations and some people evoke revulsion in me.						
13-	I get hurt very easily. On such occasions I feel humiliated and degraded.						
14-	I cannot express myself fully before others. I am generally inhibited in my behaviour.						
15-	Emotionally, I am bland. I do not get disturbed even at the suffering of my near and dear ones.						
16-	I set realistic goals and pursue them with tenacity.						
17-	I have good insight into my thinking and actions and I am in complete control of my behaviour.						
18-	I never react when I am angry. I analyse each situation thoroughly when I am cool and then react.						
19-	For me two plus two is always five. I am optimistic even in face of repeated failure.						
20-	I have a positive attitude in life. I always help people whenever I can. I do not work against the interest of anyone.						

*Affirm * Confirm * Claim Your Life!*

SELF-TALK WORKSHEET
Changing From Negative to Positive

In many situations, the only thing we can control is our **own response**. Changing self-talk from negative to positive is an excellent way to manage that response and stress.

Naming
We all name our experiences. "Crisis," "bad as usual," "a great challenge" are names you might give to things that happen.
Pick a recent upsetting experience. Describe it in a few words._____
Is there a positive name you could give it? (learning experience, chance to change, etc.)_____
List the names you gave to five recent experiences, good or bad._____
If they happened to someone else, what other positive names could you give them?_____
_____

Letting Go
You often must let go of dreams, people or parts of your life. Letting go allows you to get on with your life when something is over.
Write down two things you need to let go of._____
_____
Imagine that each one is really going out of your life. How do you feel? (sad, angry, relieved, etc)_____
_____
Who can you tell about your feeling?_____
What advice would you give to someone who is in your situation?_____
_____

Belief and Faith
Self-talk reflects our belief in who we are or in the universe. A positive faith can help you during stressful times.

Name 10 positive things you believe in about yourself people or the universe. If you can't think of 10 beliefs, ask other people for theirs. _____
_____
Describe a recent experience and how you used one of these beliefs to help you. _____
_____

HOW STORYTELLING AFFECTS THE BRAIN

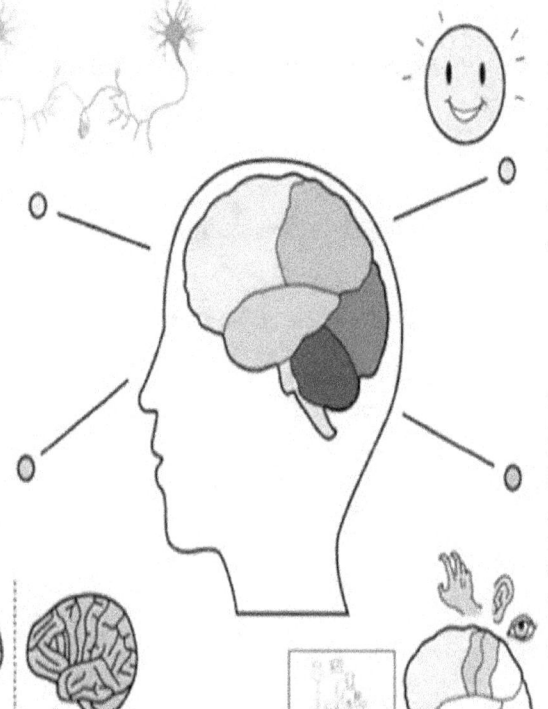

NEURAL COUPLING
A story activates parts in the brain that allows the listener to turn the story into their own ideas and experience thanks to a process called neural coupling.

DOPAMINE
The brain releases dopamine into the system when it experiences an emotionally charged event, making it easier to remember and with greater accuracy.

MIRRORING
Listeners will not only experience the similar brain activity to each other, but also to the speaker.

CORTEX ACTIVITY
When processing facts, two areas of the brain are activated (Broca's and Wernicke's area). A well-told story can engage many additional areas, including the motor cortex, sensory cortex and frontal cortex.

*Affirm * Confirm * Claim Your Life!*

Affirm!

*****

In this section we develop our THINKING about Ourselves!

We explore and utilize the best scientific and psychological concepts and research to apply to taking a Critical internal, mental examination of ourselves and create the Positive and High Energy Thoughts to complete the 'I AM' statements.

Our main purpose is to increase our ability to manifest Determined and Focused Healing, Health, Life and Power Thoughts, while being fully Cognizant and actively understanding that our thoughts are the Foundation for our Successfully Healing and Empowering!

Psychologists who study **cognition** focus on the mental activities associated with thinking, knowing, remembering, and communicating information. One of these activities is forming **concepts**—mental groupings of similar objects, events, ideas, and people.

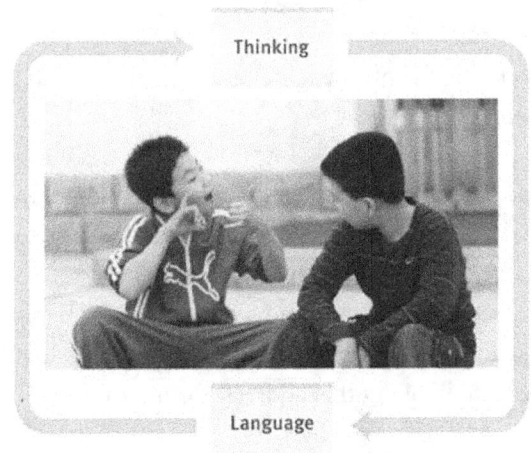

Cognition - the mental activities associated with thinking, knowing, remembering, and communicating.

Concept - a mental grouping of similar objects, events, ideas, and people.

We often form our concepts by developing a **prototype**—a mental image or best example of a category

*Affirm * Confirm * Claim Your Life!*

Prototype - a mental image or best example of a category. Matching new items to a prototype provides a quick and easy method for sorting items into categories

One tribute to our rationality is our problem-solving skill. Some problems we solve through *trial and error.*

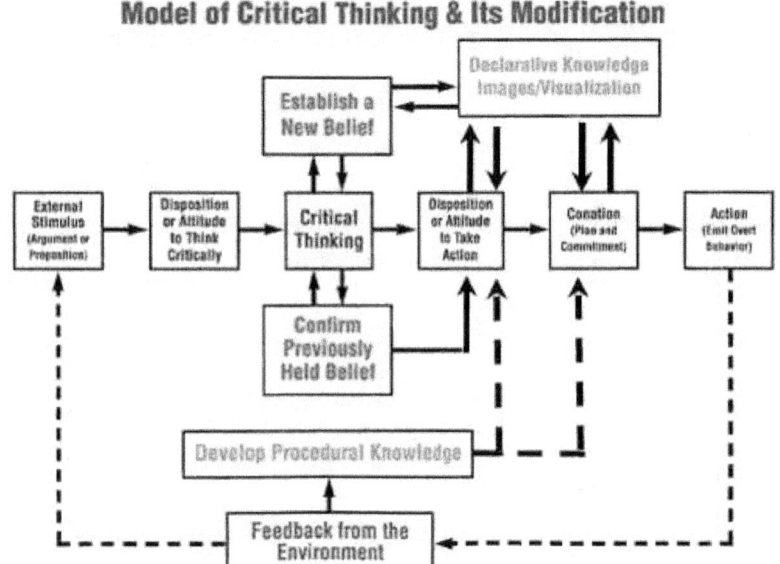

Thomas Edison tried thousands of light bulb filaments before stumbling upon one that worked. For other problems, we use **algorithms,** step-by-step procedures that guarantee a solution.

Rather than give you a computing brain the size of a beach ball, nature resorts to **heuristics,** simpler thinking strategies.

Algorithm - a methodical, logical rule or procedure that guarantees solving a particular problem. Contrasts with the usually speedier—but also more error-prone—use of *heuristics.*

Heuristic - a simple thinking strategy that often allows us to make judgments and solve problems efficiently; usually speedier but also more error prone than *algorithms.*

We will use both heuristics and algorithm to form simple and complex thoughts to complete the 'I AM' statements. We have to produce thoughts about our total Self – Mind, Body and Soul. We have to create thinking that addresses our surface level as well as going to the root of our Humanity – GOD!

Sometimes we puzzle over a problem and the pieces suddenly fall together in a flash of **insight**—an abrupt, true-seeming, and often satisfying solution (Topolinski & Reber, 2010). Unfortunately, for many of us, our own Lives are a puzzle.

Affirm * Confirm * Claim Your Life!

If we have never looked at ourselves beyond the definition of ourselves that was given to us or created by others. This leaves a lot of us STUCK and NOT knowing WHO we are and/or HOW to express ourselves.

Insight - a sudden realization of a problem's solution; contrasts with strategy-based solutions.

Teams of researchers have identified brain activity associated with sudden flashes of insight (Kounios & Beeman, 2009; Sandkühler & Bhattacharya, 2008). They gave people a problem: Think of a word that will form a compound word or phrase with each of three other words in a set (such as *pine, crab,* and *sauce*), and press a button to sound a bell when you know the answer.

(If you need a hint: The word is a fruit.?[2]) EEGs or fMRIs (functional MRIs) revealed the problem solvers' brain activity. In the first experiment, about half the solutions were by a sudden Aha! insight. Before the Aha! moment, the problem solvers' frontal lobes (which are involved in focusing attention) were active, and there was a burst of activity in the right temporal lobe, just above the ear

A burst of right temporal lobe EEG activity accompanied insight solutions to word problems (Jung-Beeman et al., 2004).

The red dots designate EEG electrodes.

The white lines show the distribution of high-frequency activity accompanying insight. The insight-related activity is centered in the right temporal lobe (yellow area).

Insight strikes suddenly, with no prior sense of "getting warmer" or feeling close to a solution (Knoblich & Oellinger, 2006; Metcalfe, 1986). When the answer pops into mind *(apple!)*, we feel a happy sense of satisfaction.

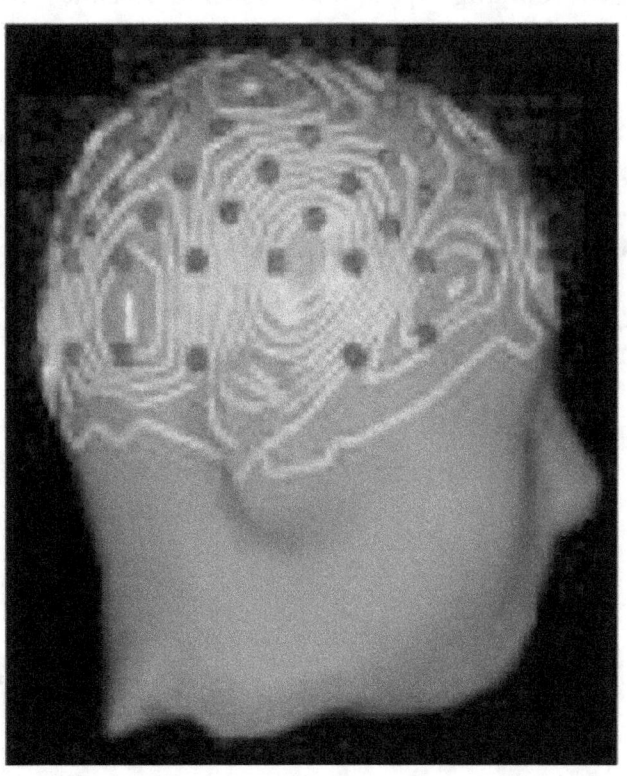

Affirm * Confirm * Claim Your Life!

The joy of a joke may similarly lie in our sudden comprehension of an unexpected ending or a double meaning: "You don't need a parachute to skydive. You only need a parachute to skydive twice."

Insightful as we are, other cognitive tendencies may lead us astray. For example, we more eagerly seek out and favor evidence that supports our ideas than evidence that refutes them (Klayman & Ha, 1987; Skov & Sherman, 1986).

Confirmation bias a tendency to search for information that supports our preconceptions and to ignore or distort contradictory evidence.

Creativity is the ability to produce ideas that are both novel and valuable (Hennessey & Amabile, 2010).

Convergent thinking narrows the available problem solutions to determine the single best solution.

Divergent thinking expands the number of possible problem solutions (creative thinking that diverges in different directions).

Personal Development Action Plan

In order to reach your goals what behaviours will you STOP, MINIMISE, KEEP DOING, do MORE of and which will you START?

	STOP	MINIMISE	KEEP DOING	Do MORE	START
1					
2					
3					
4					
5					

Affirm * Confirm * Claim Your Life!

VISUALIZATION - Mental Picturing the God that IS SELF!

We are Created with the Ability to Produce a Mental Picture/Visualization and Manifest that Mental Picture/Visualization in REALITY.

The Level of Concentration & the Quality of Our PHYSICAL Self is the Catalyst between bringing that Level Visualization & Abilities to bring it INTO Reality..

A Thought is Developed into a Mental Picture = WHAT we can Visualize we can make Manifest.

The Brain is the Control Center of Self. The Health of the Brain is the Catalyst between being able to VISUALIZE & the Quality of the Mental Picture.

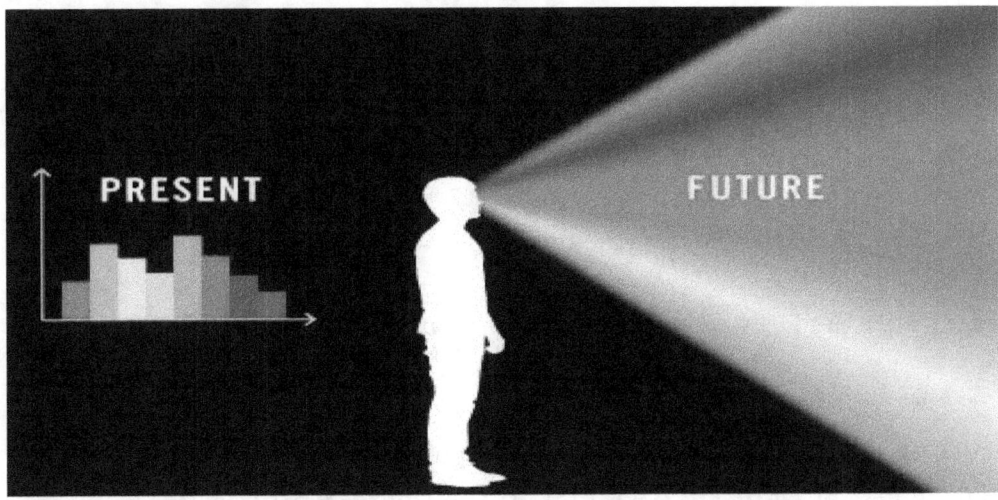

PRAYER & FASTING are the best ways to Strengthen the Mind & Produce the Highest Quality Thoughts.

GOD is the Highest Quality of ENERGY/VIBRATION/LIFE..

PRAYER/Thoughts of God elevates the Energy/Vibration Level in Self = the Ability to Produce the Highest quality Thoughts = Drawing Righteous Mental Pictures/Visualizations = BUILDING HEAVEN OVER-NIGHT !

Affirm * Confirm * Claim Your Life!

THOUGHTS are the Foundation for Developing Visualizations/Mental Pictures.

Every THOUGHT produces an Equal Corresponding CHEMICAL HORMONE.

The Higher Quality Thoughts = Stronger the Chemical Hormones = Maximum Force & Power to make Manifest the Thoughts.

What & How we Eat determines the Health of the PITUITARY Gland (Master Gland) which Signals the Corresponding CHEMICAL HORMONE to go with the Thought.

An Under Nourished PITUITARY Gland = Weakened Signal to Produce Corresponding CHEMICAL HORMONE to make Manifest the Thought.

The Chemical Hormones that Circulate the Thought thru Self are Nutrition Dependent.

A Healthy Self = Strong Chemical Hormones = Maximum Power to make Manifest the Thought..

ANYTHING that we want in Life begins as a Thought.

We Build that Thought up into a Visualization/Mental Picture.

Concentration on that Visualization produces a Steady Flow of Chemical Hormones that ARE that Visualization.

The Longer the Duration of Concentration = The Longer the Corresponding CHEMICAL HORMONE Circulates thru Self = BECOMING THAT VISUALIZATION = ABILITY TO MANIFEST THAT VISUALIZATION INTO REALITY..!

We Want To HEAL OurSelves!

Produce the Thought of Healing YourSelf...BUILD on that THOUGHT by Mentally Picturing/Visualizing Self and What and Where You Need Healing ….... Concentrate on that Visual……… Visualize Your Body producing the Corresponding CHEMICAL HORMONES of HEALING Circulating thru Self...   Visualize Self BECOMING HEALED ……... BE HEALED!

Supreme Health & Fitness!   *Knowledge Of Self Series Vol 2!*

Affirm * Confirm * Claim Your Life!

We Want POWER!

Produce the Thought of Being POWERFFUL ……..BUILD on that THOUGHT by Mentally Picturing/Visualizing Self as BEING POWERFUL ……... Concentrate on that Visual………. Visualize YourSelf producing the Corresponding CHEMICAL HORMONES of POWER Circulating thru Self ……... Visualize Self BECOMING POWERFUL …... BE POWERFUL!

We are Created in the Direct Express Image & Likeness of GOD!

Produce the Thought of Self BEING the Image & Likeness of GOD... Build that THOUGHT into a Visualization/Mental Picture of Self BEING that Image & Likeness..... Visualize the Corresponding CHEMICAL HORMONES of Self BEING GOD Circulate thru Self... Visualize Self BECOMING God.... BE GOD!

Visualize a Peaceful Life

Your mind might be addicted to negative thinking, most minds are. You will have to consciously break out of this addiction if you want to attract positive energy within you. Stay conscious and see your mind churning out fearful images. Stop thinking these thoughts and focus your attention on visualizing a peaceful flow of life. You will be amazed at the positive vibes you feel in your body.

*Affirm * Confirm * Claim Your Life!*

BENEATH THE THINKING CAP
The Basic Functions of the Brain

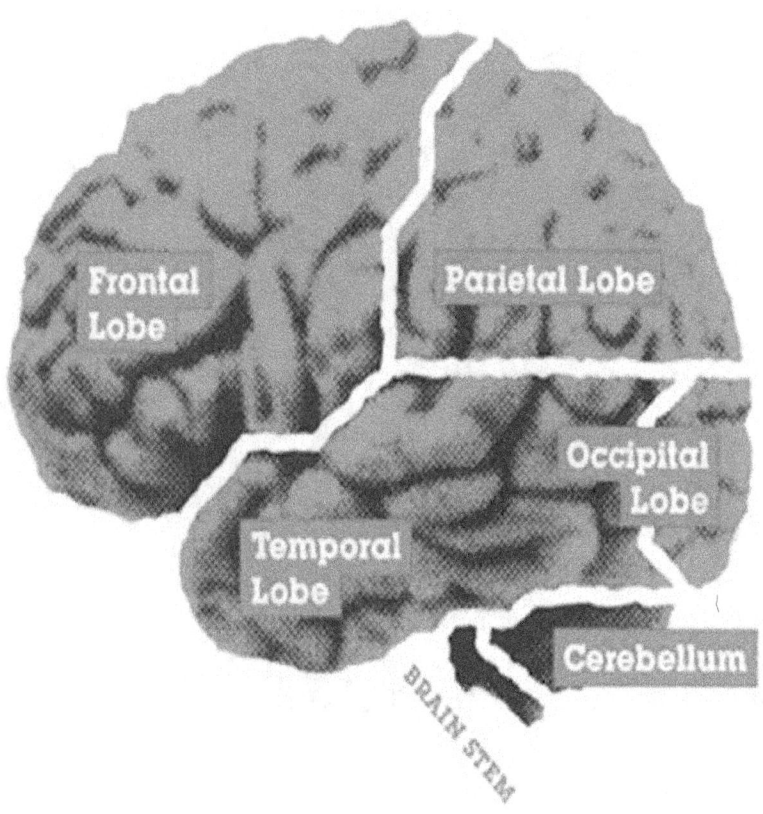

This is your brain.

It's made up of over 100 billion neurons packed into squishy folds with the consistency of tofu. At just three pounds, it barely tips the scales ahead of a pineapple. Despite its frequent use and necessity for life, the brain is a thick, mysterious forest, with a standard theory yet to come on brain function.

*Affirm * Confirm * Claim Your Life!*

IMPROVE THE MOMENT WORKSHEET
ADVANCED DISTRESS TOLERANCE SKILLS

IMAGERY

1. **WHEN RUMINATING ABOUT THE PAST**
   a. Remember & LIST times/things you did you're proud of or at which you were successful.
      - _____
      - _____
      - _____
   b. Remember & LIST any good memories or people from your past who were kind/helpful.
      - _____
      - _____
      - _____
   c. Safe Place (describe) _____

   FLASHBACKS
   a. When having flashbacks, imagine each memory:
      - being encased in a balloon and, when you pop the balloon, the flashback explodes.
      - being encased in a piñata. When you break the piñata, what will come out of it? _____
   b. When having flashbacks:
      1. Imagine yourself shrinking the images and memories that come into your head and then picking them up and putting them in a tiny box & burning it or in a bottle.
      2. Imagine changing the colors in the images to black & white.
      3. Imagine making the images out of focus or turning them upside down.
      4. Imagine turning the volume down or increasing the speed to chipmunk speed.
   c. When having flashbacks:
      - Imagine yourself surrounded by the police, army, or whatever forces you need to be in control of this memory and make things happen in your imagination the way you wished it could have happened years ago. Who would you bring with you & what would they do?
      _____
      _____

2. **WHEN RUMINATING ABOUT THE FUTURE**
   a. Play the positive "What if…" Game and imagine good things happening.
      - What if _____ [something good] happened?
      - What if _____ [everything turned out better than I hoped]?
      - Ask what am I able to do now? What is needed? Let go of the impossible.
   b. IMAGINE (Yourself as a superhero able to "save the day" and vanquish all the bad guys).
      - What super powers would you have? _____.
      - What would your "Super" name be? _____.
      - What kind of costume would you wear? _____.
   c. What if you over-extended your catastrophizing & imagined adding lots of silly things to the story your mind is trying to tell you?
   d. What if your wildest & best fantasy came true? What would happen?

Supreme Health & Fitness! Knowledge Of Self Series Vol 2!

*Affirm * Confirm * Claim Your Life!*

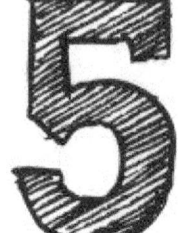 THINGS THAT I LIKE ABOUT MYSELF...

1) _____

2) _____

3) _____

4) _____

5) _____

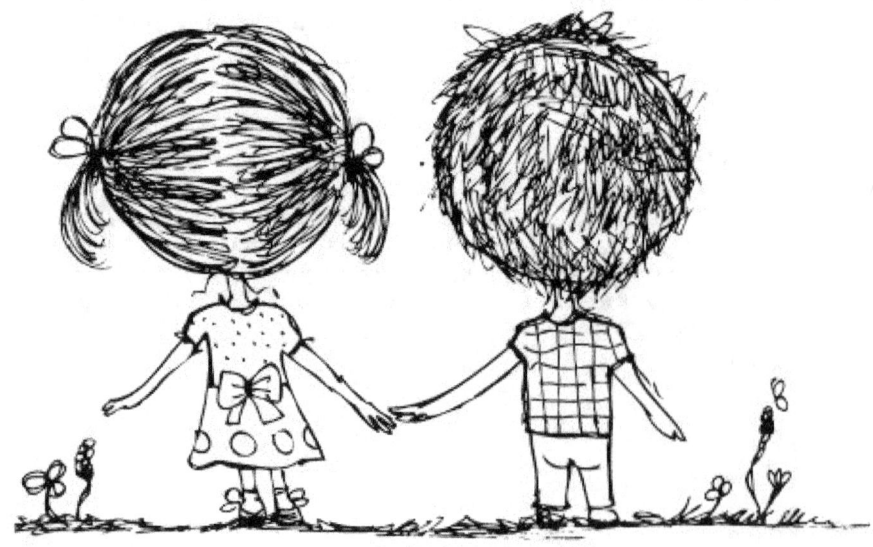

Affirm * Confirm * Claim Your Life!

Life Story
The Past, Present, and Future

Writing a story about your life can help you find meaning and value in your experiences. It will allow you to organize your thoughts and use them to grow. People who develop stories about their life tend to experience a greater sense of meaning, which can contribute to happiness.

The Past
Write the story of your past. Be sure to describe challenges you've overcome, and the personal strengths that allowed you to do so.

_____

_____

_____

_____

_____

_____

_____

_____

_____

_____

_____

_____

_____

_____

*Affirm * Confirm * Claim Your Life!*

Speak Life!

I Matter • I Am Loved • I Can Make It

I'm Hanging In There • I Will Not Give Up

I Am Blessed • I Am A Winner

I Am More Than A Conqueror

I Have Favor With God and With Man

God's Gonna Get The Glory Out of This

I Am Strong • I Am Healed • I Am Whole

I Can Do This • Yes I Can • Read: Proverbs 18:21

Affirm * Confirm * Claim Your Life!

YOUR VOICE COMMANDS YOUR MIND, BODY & SPIRIT

Learn the true meaning of each word, the root and the original intention. Find the cousins to each word, say it, feel it, which one will move you forward in your own life?

ENERGY + VIBRATION = MATTER

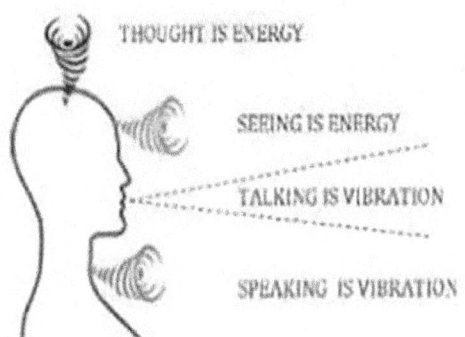

THOUGHTS + VOICE = REALITY

Help the self by Walking the Absolute Truth of your own life, Meditate & Pray...Keep thoughts, actions & words positive...Be self empowered and use the tools presented in a good way

Made with unconditional love,
Barbara M. Moreau, Angel who dances on the Clouds
Frank J. Austin, Manyhorses (Teacher)

I can't I won't It's hard I Don't Believe I'm a skeptic I don't like it	=	• Will literally stop growth • Will literally put a block in your way • Can not is a command to self • Will literally stop you from achieving anything in your life • Is a taught behavior that is a conditional to hold a person back • Stops a person from learning • Stops a person from gaining intellect (IQ)
Try Trying I can try I'm trying I will try I will attempt	=	• Try and you will do it over and over and over never get to the end • Puts a block in your way • Try is a command to self • Try and trying is a taught behavior that is a condition to hold a person back • It has very little or no results • It is like running a race with no end • It is never ending • It is repetitious
I can I am I believe It is done I can do it I can do anything	=	• Literally promotes growth • Can is a command to self • Allows your wants, needs and desire to come true • Is a behavior of using good words • It is unconditional and moves a person forward in life • When you know inside you can do it your body needs to hear it • Your body reacts to key words

Supreme Health & Fitness!   Knowledge Of Self Series Vol 2!

Affirm * Confirm * Claim Your Life!

Wait A Minute—
Aren't You Made Up Of Water?

Yes! 72% of your body is made up of water. Imagine how your words affect your own body. When you say, "I'm a failure," or "I'm hopeless," or "I won't get well," imagine how these words weaken your health.
Make a choice to say the best words out there.
Say often, "I'm wonderful," "I'm beautiful," "I'm God's child," and "God has a great plan for my life!"

I AM _____!

I AM _____!

I AM _____!

I AM _____!

I AM _____!

I AM _____!

I AM _____!

Affirm * Confirm * Claim Your Life!

I AM _____!

I AM _____!

I AM _____!

I AM _____!

I AM _____!

I AM _____!

I AM _____!

I AM _____!

I AM _____!

I AM _____!

I AM _____!

I AM _____!

I AM _____!

I AM _____!

I AM _____!

Affirm * Confirm * Claim Your Life!

I AM _____!

I AM _____!

I AM _____!

"Today is an incredible day! Success, Prosperity, and Abundance, in many different forms have naturally found their way into my life today. I gratefully enjoy their manifestations throughout my day and happily share these blessings of abundance with many others in order to bring happiness to their day as well."

"I Am Happy"
"I Am Healthy"
"I Am Wealthy"
"I Am Secure"
"I Am Worthy"
"I Am Positive"
"I Am Blessed"
"I Am Grateful"
"I Am Beautiful"
"I Am Confident"
"I Am Courageous"
"I Am Excited About Today"
"I Am Loved"

*Affirm * Confirm * Claim Your Life!*

I CAN _____!

I CAN _____!

I CAN _____!

I CAN _____!

I CAN _____!

I CAN _____!

I CAN _____!

I CAN _____!

I CAN _____!

I CAN _____!

I CAN _____!

I CAN _____!

I CAN _____!

I CAN _____!

Affirm * Confirm * Claim Your Life!

I CAN _____!

I CAN _____!

I CAN _____!

I CAN _____!

I CAN _____!

I CAN _____!

I CAN _____!

I CAN _____!

I CAN _____!

I CAN _____!

I CAN _____!

I CAN _____!

I CAN _____!

I CAN _____!

I CAN _____!

Affirm * Confirm * Claim Your Life!

I WILL _____!

I WILL _____!

I WILL _____!

I WILL _____!

I WILL _____!

I WILL _____!

I WILL _____!

I WILL _____!

I WILL _____!

I WILL _____!

I WILL _____!

I WILL _____!

I WILL _____!

I WILL _____!

*Affirm * Confirm * Claim Your Life!*

I WILL _____!

I WILL _____!

I WILL _____!

I WILL _____!

I WILL _____!

I WILL _____!

I WILL _____!

I WILL _____!

I WILL _____!

I WILL _____!

I WILL _____!

I WILL _____!

I WILL _____!

I WILL _____!

When you declare "I am
OPEN

and ready to receive"

The universe not only hears you, it holds out its hands to help you.

*Affirm * Confirm * Claim Your Life!*

MIND, BODY AND SPIRIT.

WEEKLY WELLNESS PLAN:
DATE: _____

TAKE CARE OF THE WHOLE YOU. ▶▶▶▶▶

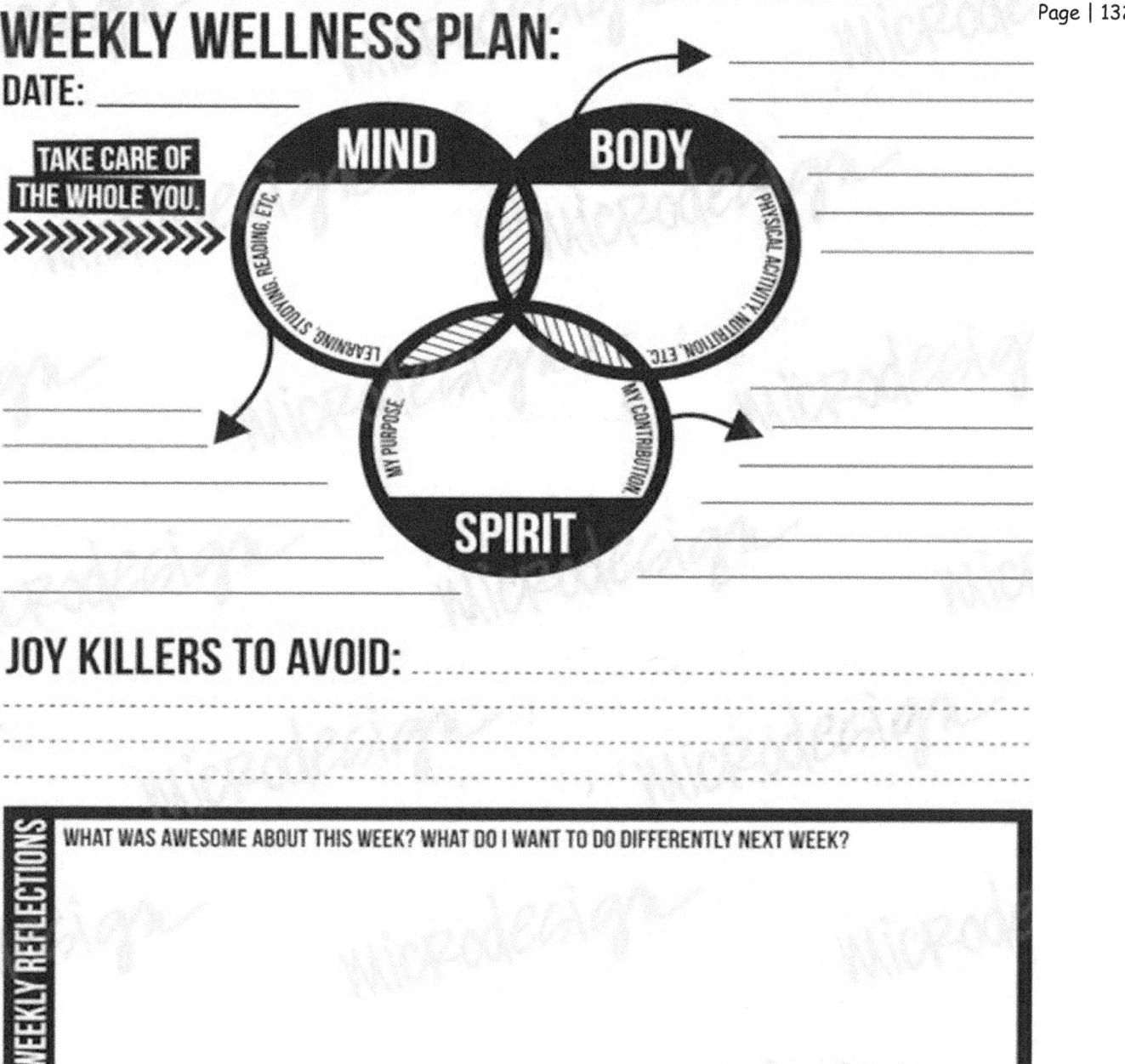

JOY KILLERS TO AVOID: ....
....
....

WEEKLY REFLECTIONS — WHAT WAS AWESOME ABOUT THIS WEEK? WHAT DO I WANT TO DO DIFFERENTLY NEXT WEEK?

Affirm * Confirm * Claim Your Life!

How Heart Activity Affects Our Ability to Think

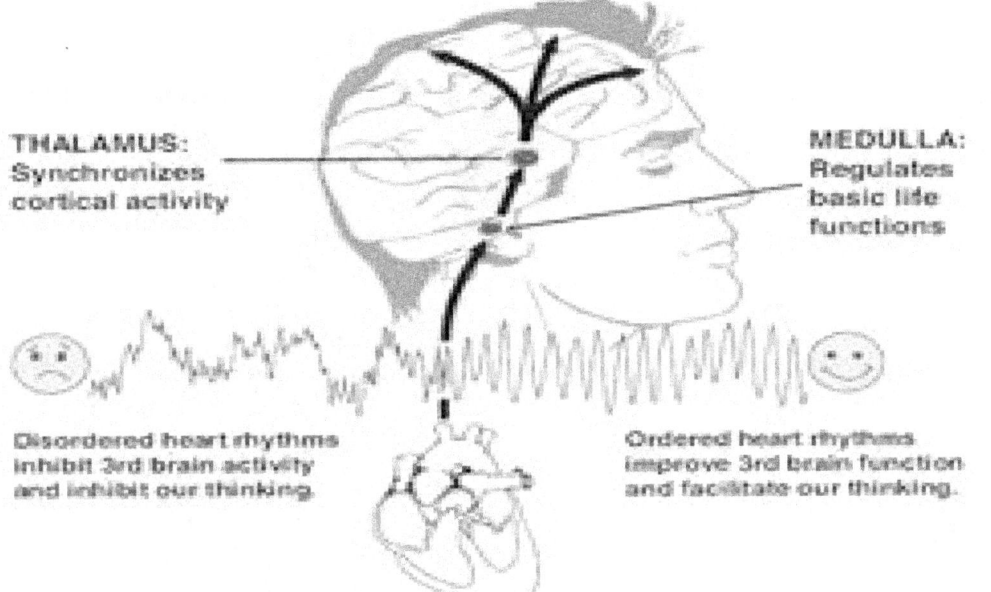

THALAMUS: Synchronizes cortical activity

MEDULLA: Regulates basic life functions

Disordered heart rhythms inhibit 3rd brain activity and inhibit our thinking.

Ordered heart rhythms improve 3rd brain function and facilitate our thinking.

What is Self Awareness ?

- "Self-awareness" refers to the capacity to become the object of one's own attention.
- It occurs when an organism focuses not on the external environment, but on the internal milieu;
- It becomes a reflective observer, processing *self-information.*
- *The organism becomes aware* that it is awake and actually experiencing specific mental events, emitting behaviors, and possessing unique characteristics.

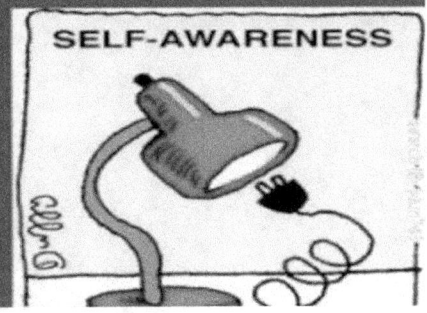

A 2009 report from Sweden's Lund University put forward six psychological mechanisms through which emotions may be produced when the brain reacts to sound.

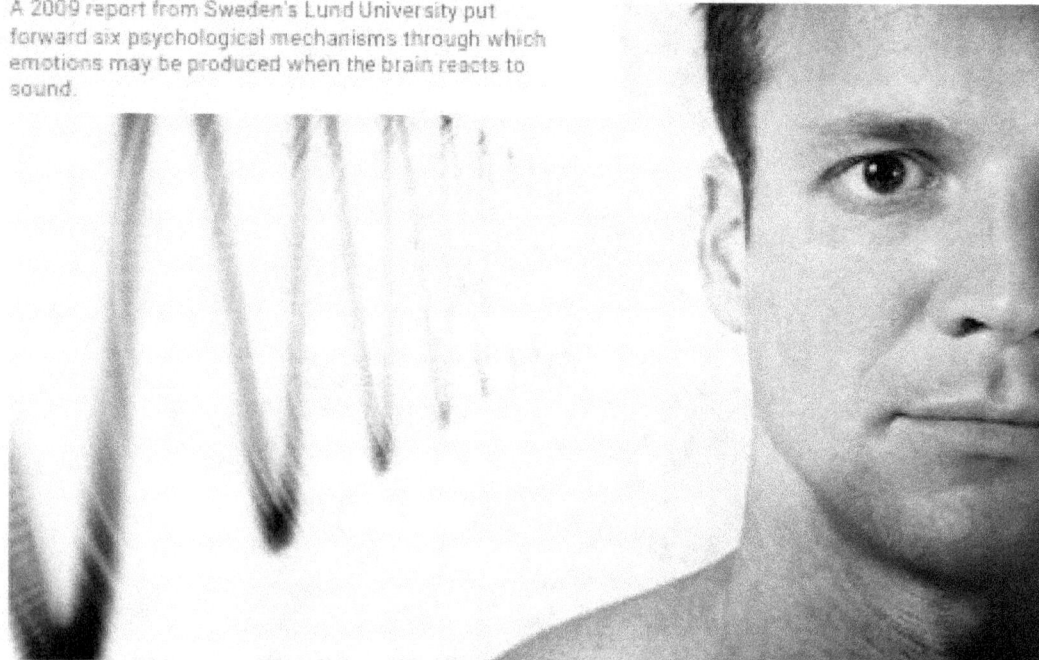

1) **Brain stem reflex:** When the acoustic characteristics of the sound (eg loud or dissonant) signal a "potentially important and urgent event", causing us to react on an instinctive level.

2) **Evaluative conditioning:** When an emotion is elicited by sound because we have heard it repeatedly in a certain setting, leading to an association between sound and setting.

3) **Emotional contagion:** When we perceive the emotion expressed by a piece of music: the music doesn't necessarily sound sad, but rather we recognise it as expressing sadness.

4) **Visual imagery:** When the structure of a piece of music makes us imagine certain scenes or sensations, such as a rising melody connecting with the sensation of moving upwards.

5) **Episodic memory:** Also known as the 'Darling, they're playing our tune' phenomenon - when a particular sound or piece of music evokes a powerful memory.

6) **Music expectancy:** This is tied to our experiences with music: for instance, an unfamiliar variation on a standard note progression like may cause feelings of surprise and curiosity.

Of these mechanisms, the authors stated that the first two are in-born reactions, the second two develop during the first few years of our lives, and the last two tend to be learned during childhood and later life.

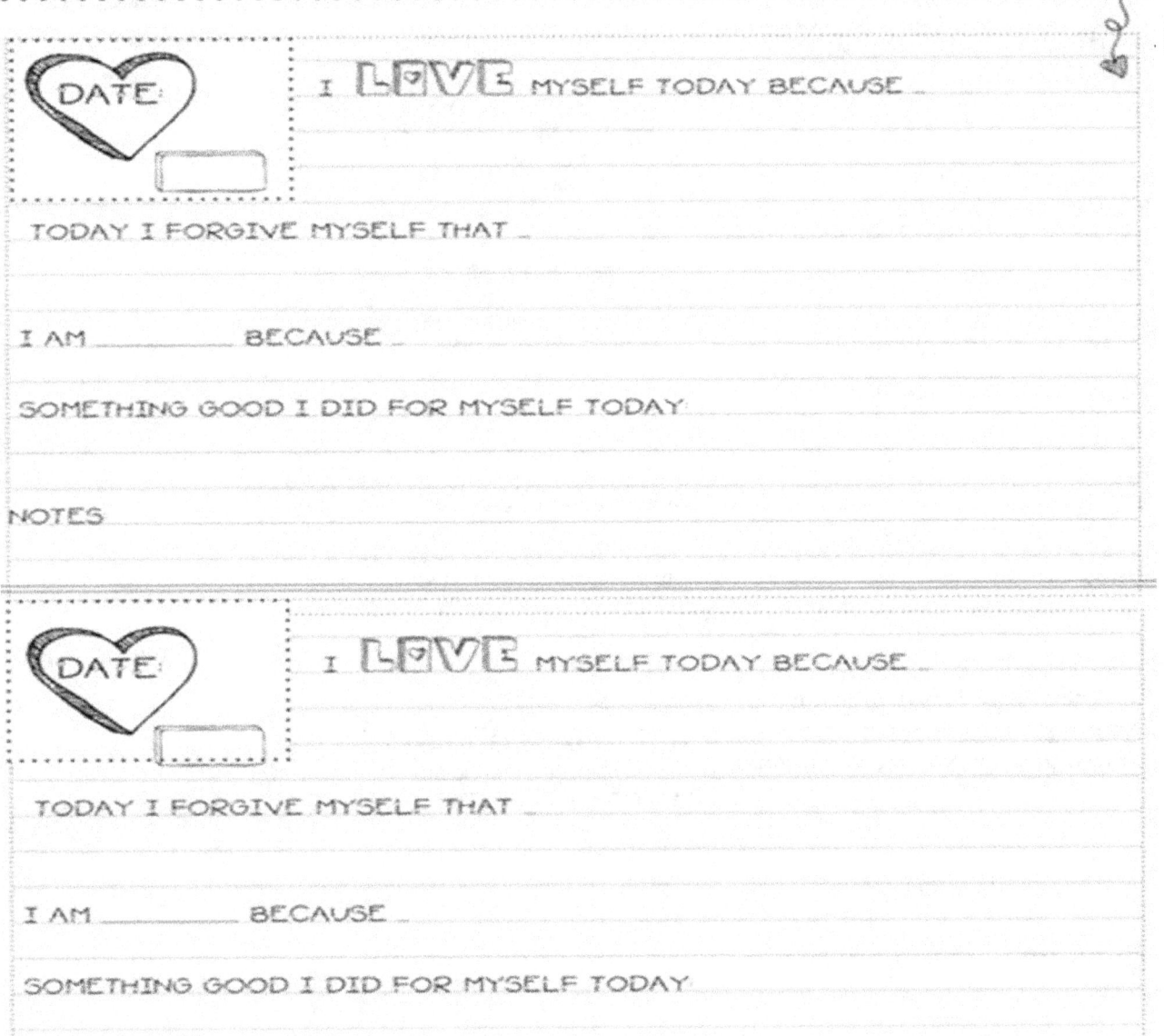

Affirm * Confirm * Claim Your Life!

1
I am fighting hard for the things I want most
- The longer you have to wait for something, the more you will appreciate it when it finally arrives.
- Most great things don't come easy, but they are worth waiting for and fighting for.

2
I am taking action now
- Many great things can be done in a day if you don't always make that day tomorrow.

3
I am focusing on the next positive step
- The future holds nothing but endless potential.
- There are far, far better things ahead than any we leave behind.

4
I am proud to wear my truth
- How you see yourself means everything.
- To be beautiful means to live confidently in your own skin.

5
I have a lot to smile about
- Happiness is not a result of getting something you don't have, but rather of recognizing and appreciating what you do have.

6
I am making the best of it
- Everything you go through grows you.
- Amazing things can and do happen when you least expect them.

7
I am letting go of yesterday's stress
- Leave behind the stress, the drama and the worries. Lay this day to rest.
- Tomorrow is about hope, new possibilities, and the opportunity to make a better day.

8
There is enough time today to do something I love
- You will find happiness in doing the thing you love to do.

9
I am priceless in someone's eyes
- Focus on those who love and accept you for who you are, and shower them with the love and kindness they deserve. Cherish the people who saw you when you were invisible to everyone else.

10
It's not too late
- No matter who you are, no matter what you did, no matter where you've come from, you can always change and become a better version of yourself.

Self-reflection is a humbling process. It's essential to find out why you think, say, and do certain things... then better yourself.

List of Coping Thoughts

Here is a list of some coping thoughts that many people have found to be helpful (McKay, Davis, & Fanning, 1997). Check (✓) the ones that are helpful to you and create your own.

- ____ "This situation won't last forever."
- ____ "I've already been through many other painful experiences, and I've survived."
- ____ "This too shall pass."
- ____ "My feelings make me uncomfortable right now, but I can accept them."
- ____ "I can be anxious and still deal with the situation."
- ____ "I'm strong enough to handle what's happening to me right now."
- ____ "This is an opportunity for me to learn how to cope with my fears."
- ____ "I can ride this out and not let it get to me."
- ____ "I can take all the time I need right now to let go and relax."
- ____ "I've survived other situations like this before, and I'll survive this one too."
- ____ "My anxiety/fear/sadness won't kill me; it just doesn't feel good right now."
- ____ "These are just my feelings, and eventually they'll go away."
- ____ "It's okay to feel sad/anxious/afraid sometimes."
- ____ "My thoughts don't control my life, I do."
- ____ "I can think different thoughts if I want to."
- ____ "I'm not in danger right now."
- ____ "So what?"
- ____ "This situation sucks, but it's only temporary."
- ____ "I'm strong and I can deal with this."
- ____ Other ideas: _____

Affirm * Confirm * Claim Your Life!

Confirm!

* * * * *

The process of Confirming our Affirmations involves Looking at ourselves and Verbally Communicate them to ourselves.

Just as with Writing, when we Talk, this is a voluntary Motion and Deliberate.

We have to produce the Electro-Chemical impulse that causes the Muscle contractions in our Mouth, Vocal Chords and Tongue to produce the corresponding Words.

When you are alone, do you talk to yourself? Is "thinking" simply conversing with your-self?

Words do convey ideas and ideas precede words.

So, with the Confirm stage, we are taking our "I AM' statements and turning them into ACTIONS!

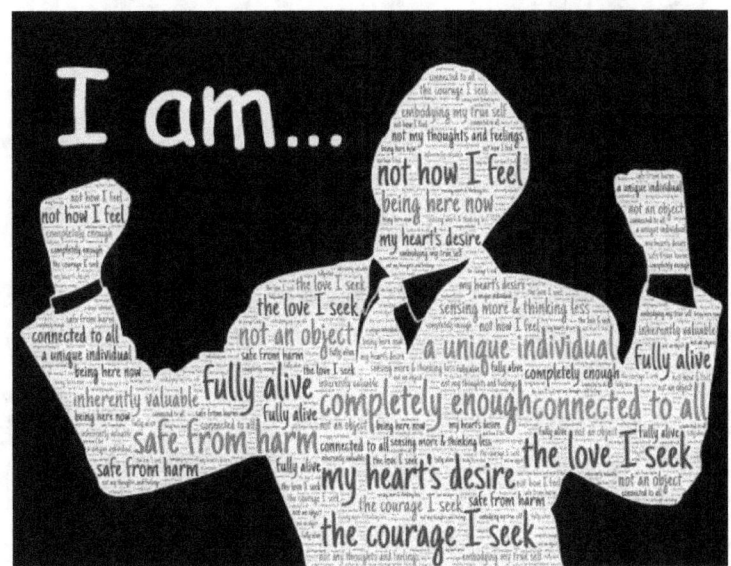

The first step is to convert the Energy of the 'I AM' statements and address yourself from a 3rd person perspective. THAT'S RIGHT …… this is your opportunity to begin the reinforcement of your Power of yourself.

So, you look at yourself from an outside perspective. You address yourself and communicate with yourself from an outside perspective. You internalize and examine yourself from an outside perspective. You Appreciate yourself from an outside perspective.

Affirm * Confirm * Claim Your Life!

This allows you to fully comprehend and Visualize yourself in the frame of all the wonderful attributive 'I AM' statements that you formed of yourself.

Energy cannot be destroyed ….. it can only be transferred and/or transformed. The 'I AM' statements are HIGH ENERGY words and we want to transform this Energy into even HIGHER forms by using the 3rd person Language.

Example – Sean, You ARE Intelligent!   Sean, You ARE Healthy!   Sean, You ARE Powerful!   Sean, You ARE Beautiful!

The Act of Writing the 'I AM' statements into 'You ARE' statements is the first step. It is changing the original thought into an Actual Reality. First you Thought, next You transformed your un-seen thought into a Seen Reality by Writing them down. Then you SPEAK your thoughts into Existence – bringing them to LIFE IN YOU!!!!!

> Proverbs 12:18 "There is one whose rash words are like sword thrusts, but the tongue of the wise brings healing."

Understanding Language

When we speak, our brain and voice apparatus conjure up air-pressure waves that we send banging against another's eardrum—enabling us to transfer thoughts from our brain into theirs.

As cognitive scientist Steven Pinker (1998) has noted, we sometimes sit for hours "listening to other people make noise as they exhale, because those hisses and squeaks contain *information*."

And thanks to all those funny sounds created in our heads from the air-pressure waves we send out, we get people's attention, we get them to do things, and we maintain relationships (Guerin, 2003).

Affirm * Confirm * Claim Your Life!

Depending on how you vibrate the air after opening your mouth, you may get slapped or kissed.

But **language** is more than vibrating air. As I create this paragraph, my fingers on a keyboard generate electronic binary numbers that are translated into the squiggles in front of you.

When transmitted by reflected light rays into your retina, those squiggles trigger formless nerve impulses that project to several areas of your brain, which integrate the information, compare it to stored information, and decode meaning.

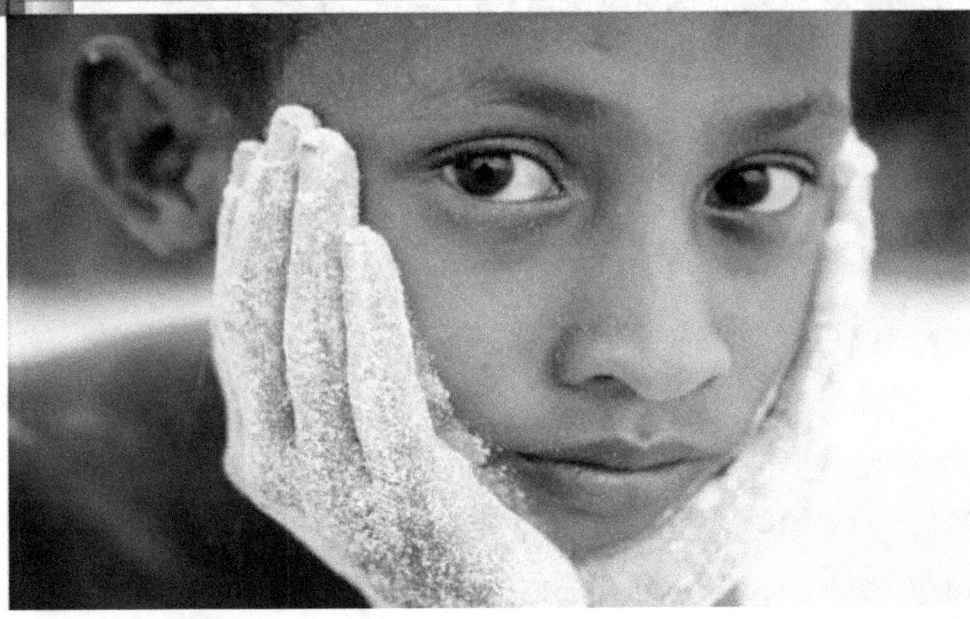

Imagine how your Own Words affect your Own Body. When you say, "I'm a failure," or "I'm hopeless," or "I won't get well," or "I cant do this"
Imagine how these Words weaken your Own Health.

The Power of Words over Water

Thanks to language, information is moving from my mind to yours. Monkeys mostly know what they see.

Thanks to language (spoken, written, or signed), we comprehend much that we've never seen and that our distant ancestors never knew.

Affirm * Confirm * Claim Your Life!

If you were able to retain only one cognitive ability, make it language, suggests researcher Lera Boroditsky (2009). Without sight or hearing, you could still have friends, family, and a job. But without language, could you have these things?

"Language is so fundamental to our experience, so deeply a part of being human, that it's hard to imagine life without it."

The most critical Language skill is the ability to effectively communicate with Self!

the power of words can move you to tears, evoke absolute joy or lead you in action. there are words of encouragement, of sympathy, of love & admiration. the right words can give you strength, define your faith, give flight to things that live in your imagination. Words will inspire you, cut you, bring you back to life. They will comfort you in your time of need. words will **nourish your soul.**

For a *spoken* language, we would need three building blocks:

- **Phonemes** are the smallest distinctive sound units in a language. To say *bat*, English speakers utter the phonemes *b, a,* and *t*. (Phonemes aren't the same as letters. *Chat* also has three phonemes—*ch, a,* and *t*.)

Linguists surveying nearly 500 languages have identified 869 different phonemes in human speech, but no language uses all of them (Holt, 2002; Maddieson, 1984). English uses about 40; other languages use anywhere from half to more than twice that many.

As a general rule, consonant phonemes carry more information than do vowel phonemes. *The treth ef thes stetement shed be evedent frem thes bref demenstretien.*

Phoneme - in a language, the smallest distinctive sound unit.

- **Morphemes** are the smallest units that carry meaning in a given language. In English, a few morphemes are also phonemes—the personal pronoun *I* and the article *a,* for instance. But most morphemes combine two or more phonemes. Some, like *bat,* are words. Others—like the prefix *pre-* in *preview* or the suffix *-ed* in *adapted*—are parts of words.

Morpheme - in a language, the smallest unit that carries meaning; may be a word or a part of a word (such as a prefix).

- **Grammar** is the system of rules that enables us to communicate with one another. Grammatical rules guide us in deriving meaning from sounds *(semantics)* and in ordering words into sentences *(syntax)*.

Grammar - in a language, a system of rules that enables us to communicate with and understand others. In a given language, *semantics* is the set of rules for deriving meaning from sounds, and *syntax* is the set of rules for combining words into grammatically sensible sentences.

What brain areas are involved in language processing and speech?

We think of speaking and reading, or writing and reading, or singing and speaking as merely different examples of the same general ability—language. But consider this curious finding: **Aphasia,** an impairment of language, can result from damage to any of several cortical areas. Even more curious, some people with aphasia can speak fluently but cannot read (despite good vision), while others can comprehend what they read but cannot speak.

Still others can write but not read, read but not write, read numbers but not letters, or sing but not speak. These cases suggest that language is complex, and that different brain areas must serve different language functions.

Aphasia - impairment of language, usually caused by left-hemisphere damage either to Broca's area (impairing speaking) or to Wernicke's area (impairing understanding).

Indeed, in 1865, French physician Paul Broca reported that after damage to an area of the left frontal lobe (later called **Broca's area**) a person would struggle to *speak* words while still being able to sing familiar songs and comprehend speech.

Broca's area controls language expression—an area of the frontal lobe, usually in the left hemisphere, that directs the muscle movements involved in speech.

Today's neuroscience has confirmed brain activity in Broca's and Wernicke's areas during language processing. But language functions are distributed across other brain areas as well

Functional MRI scans show that what you experience as a continuous, indivisible stream of experience—language—is actually but the visible tip of a subdivided information-processing iceberg.

Different neural networks are activated by nouns and verbs (or objects and actions); by different vowels; and by reading stories of visual versus motor experiences (Shapiro et al., 2006; Speer et al., 2009).

If you are bilingual, the neural networks that enable your native language differ from those that enable your second language (Perani & Abutalebi, 2005).

In processing language, as in other forms of information processing, *the brain operates by dividing its mental functions—speaking, perceiving, thinking, remembering—into sub-functions*.

Your conscious experience of reading this page *seems* indivisible, but you are engaging many different neural networks in your brain to compute each word's form, sound, and meaning (Posner & Carr, 1992).

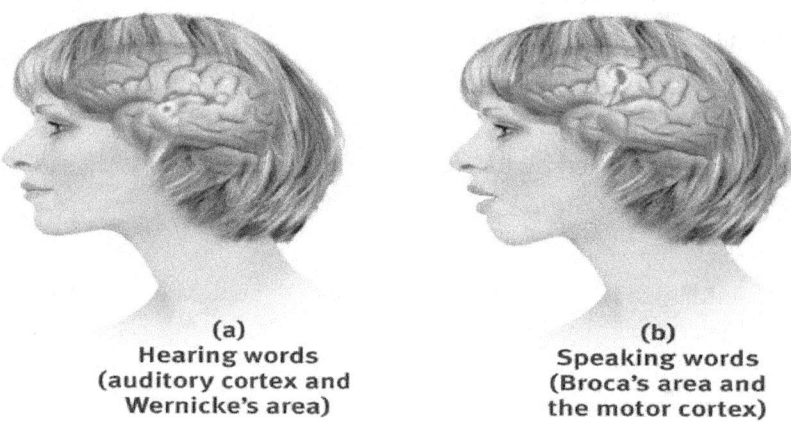

(a) Hearing words (auditory cortex and Wernicke's area)

(b) Speaking words (Broca's area and the motor cortex)

Affirm * Confirm * Claim Your Life!

What is the relationship between thinking and language, and what is the value of thinking in images?

Thinking and language intricately intertwine. Asking which comes first is one of psychology's chicken-and-egg questions. Do our ideas come first and we wait for words to name them? Or are our thoughts conceived in words and therefore unthinkable without them?

Given words' subtle influence on thinking, we do well to choose our words carefully. Does it make any difference whether I write, "I am Great" or "I can be Great"?

To expand language is to expand the ability to think

5. Use Power Words

A study at the University of California showed that the most persuasive words in spoken language are: *discovery, guarantee, love, proven, results, save, easy, health, money, new, safety* and *you*. Practise using these words. The new results you'll get from the discovery of these proven words will guarantee you more love, better health and will save you money. And they're completely safe, and easy to use.

*Affirm * Confirm * Claim Your Life!*

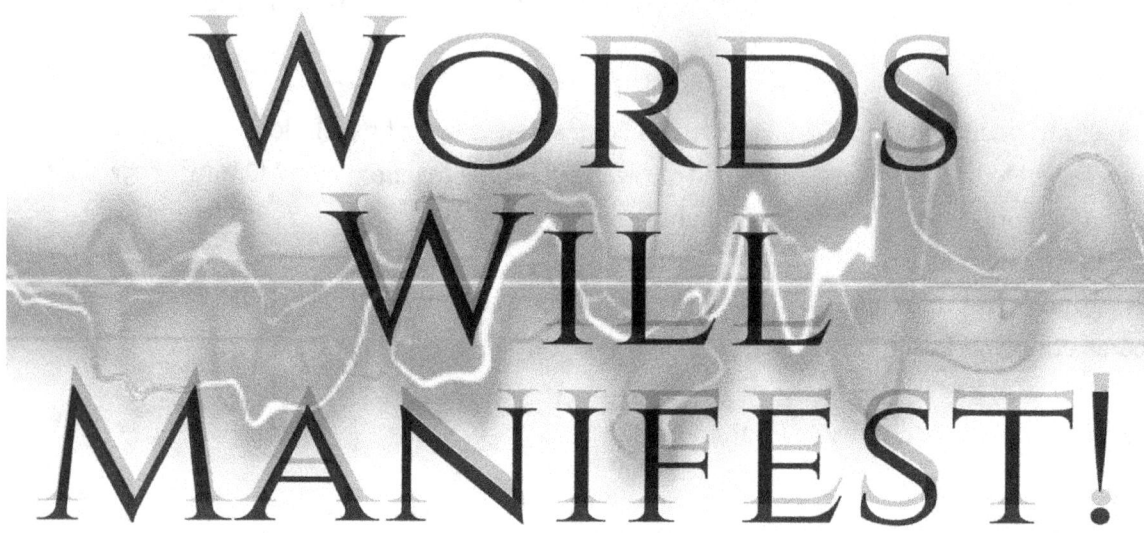

_____, You ARE _____!

_____, You ARE _____!

_____, You ARE _____!

_____, You ARE _____!

_____, You ARE _____!

_____, You ARE _____!

_____, You ARE _____!

_____, You ARE _____!

_____, You ARE _____!

_____, You ARE _____!

Affirm * Confirm * Claim Your Life!

_____, You ARE _____!

_____, You ARE _____!

_____, You ARE _____!

_____, You ARE _____!

_____, You ARE _____!

_____, You ARE _____!

_____, You ARE _____!

_____, You ARE _____!

_____, You ARE _____!

_____, You ARE _____!

_____, You ARE _____!

_____, You ARE _____!

_____, You ARE _____!

_____, You ARE _____!

_____, You ARE _____!

_____, You ARE _____!

- I accept myself as I am.
- I am enough.
- I am worthy of compassion.
- I forgive myself and allow myself to feel inner peace.
- I allow myself to make mistakes and to learn from those mistakes.
- I let go of the old and make room for the new.
- Today I will treat myself with kindness.
- Like any human being, I have strengths and weaknesses, and that's OK.
- I'm healing through self-compassion.
- I give myself the gift of unconditional love.

Affirm * Confirm * Claim Your Life!

_____, You WILL BE _____!

_____, You WILL BE _____!

_____, You WILL BE _____!

_____, You WILL BE _____!

_____, You WILL BE _____!

_____, You WILL BE _____!

_____, You WILL BE _____!

_____, You WILL BE _____!

_____, You WILL BE _____!

_____, You WILL BE _____!

_____, You WILL BE _____!

_____, You WILL BE _____!

_____, You WILL BE _____!

_____, You WILL BE _____!

_____, You WILL BE _____!

_____, You WILL BE _____!

Affirm * Confirm * Claim Your Life!

_____, You WILL BE _____!

_____, You WILL BE _____!

_____, You WILL BE _____!

_____, You WILL BE _____!

_____, You WILL BE _____!

_____, You WILL BE _____!

_____, You WILL BE _____!

_____, You WILL BE _____!

_____, You WILL BE _____!

_____, You WILL BE _____!

_____, You WILL BE _____!

_____, You WILL BE _____!

_____, You WILL BE _____!

_____, You WILL BE _____!

_____, You WILL BE _____!

_____, You WILL BE _____!

*Affirm * Confirm * Claim Your Life!*

Chapter

Power of Words On WATER – YOU!

*****

Did you know one positive word can change water's structure? Do you know that there is proof. A Japanese scientist named Masaru Emoto made a series of tests and discovered some very interesting results.

Emoto realized both positive and negative words can have an influence on water's structure by changing water's crystals.

During his study of water, Emoto came to some fascinating revelations. He came to a belief that water was the so-called ''blueprint of our reality'' and our emotional energy and vibrations can change the physical structure of water. Emoto's tests mostly consisted of putting water in glasses and then exposing it to different words, pictures, and music and then freezing it and analyzing how water crystals look. And through his research and analysis, he came to the conclusion that if we "influence" water with positive words, pictures, or music that water crystals will be nicely formed.

On the other hand, if one puts water near negative influences, such as saying negative words, or if you turn on some loud heavy metal music then the results would be the total opposite.

Those water crystals will be distorted and formed in an ugly and negative formation.

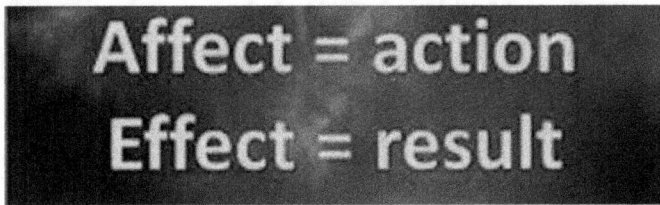

*Affirm * Confirm * Claim Your Life!*

But what happens with us when we are influenced by both positive and negative things? Do we react the same way water reacts? Does our molecule structure also change when someone says something nice to us?

The answer for that is simply — yes.

We are approximately 75% WATER and as such we are also prone to changes. Our molecule structure also changes when influenced by different words, music, movies, scenes of violence (or love), etc...... Water Absorbs and is SHAPED by its outside environment and Energy.

Words are Energy or Contain Energy ..... When we Hear Words – from ourselves or others – the Energy Shapes and Affects US – Transforming YOU INTO THOSE WORDS/ENERGY!

You will use this Science to AFFECT and EFFECT Your Healing, Life, Power and Greatness!!!

MESSAGES FROM WATER
How the molecular structure of water is affected...

Mr. Emoto's
- human, thoughts, words, ideas and music, affect the molecular structure of water,
- 70% of our human body is water
- 70% covers of our planet

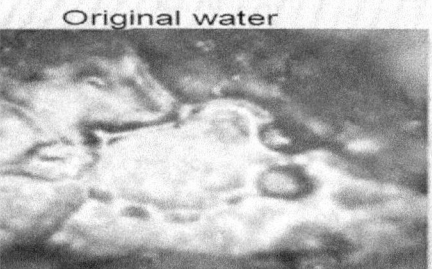
Original water

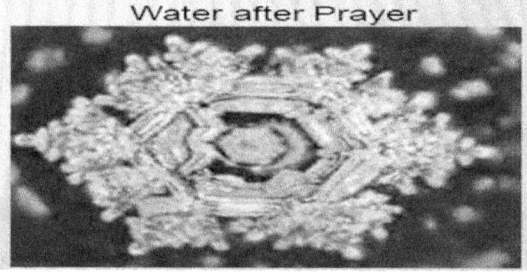
Water after Prayer

With this WorkBook, You are creating Your Own High Energy Words and Language, that when you Read and Hear them You Shape Yourself INTO them.

You Write and Read the High Energy Words of YOUR HEALING = Shape and Affect YOUR HEALING!

Affirm * Confirm * Claim Your Life!

You will create the AFFECT of the Action of Energy that will Successfully EFFECT and make Manifest YOUR HEALING!

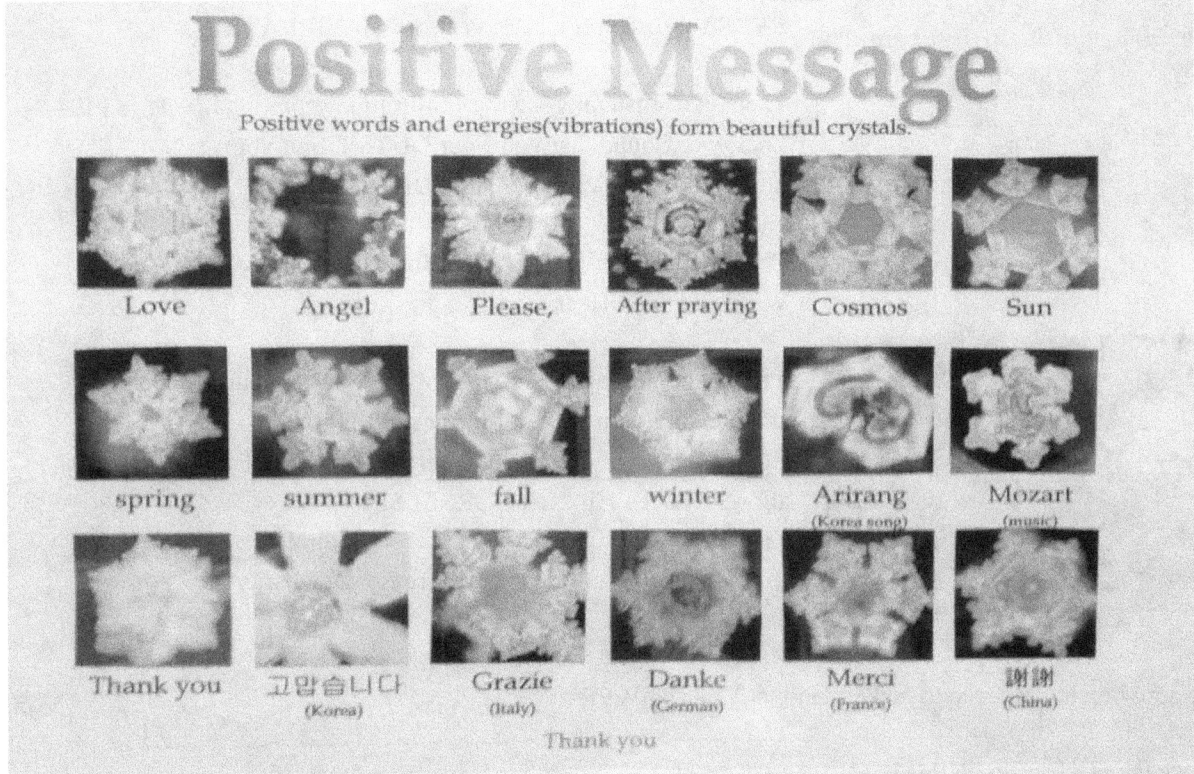

With this book, you will apply the Science of words and sounds on Water to Positively Vibrate and raise the Energy Level and Frequency of Your Water of Your Body.

By Thinking Positive High Energy words, the Foundation is laid for your Transformation INTO your Thoughts. These Thoughts create the Energy and Vibration level in you.

You reinforce and increase this energy and vibration by WRITING down your Thoughts. This is ACTION and involves You moving the Water of Your Body to physically manifest your unseen Thought.

After the Action of WRITING, now you take the Empowering Action of READING your Thoughts. The Act of Reading creates vibrations and energy IN you to is attuned to the Words you are reading. Because these are HIGH Energy words, written about Your HEALING, Life, Power and Greatness – Your further increasing the CHANGE of yourself INTO your Words.

Affirm * Confirm * Claim Your Life!

This means you are transforming the Thought of Healing INTO the ACTION of Healing!

Dr. Emoto tested water samples by writing and focusing negative words, thoughts and intentions on one set, and positive, loving intentions on the other. The results showed that bad thoughts provided ugly, unappealing water crystals. Happy thoughts in turn, created beautiful, intricate water crystals.

EVERY Word you HEAR is a form of VIBRATION.

The Act of Listening is your Eardrum interpreting the Energy or Sound that you Hear OUTSIDE of you into Energy and Vibration INSIDE YOU!

This Shapes the Water of your Body INTO the Words that you Hear.

You are beginning the Process of re-defining yourself and creating your own definitions of Self while simultaneously creating the environment IN Self that allows You To HEAL YOURSELF!

You are using this science to increase the Quality of Your LIFE!

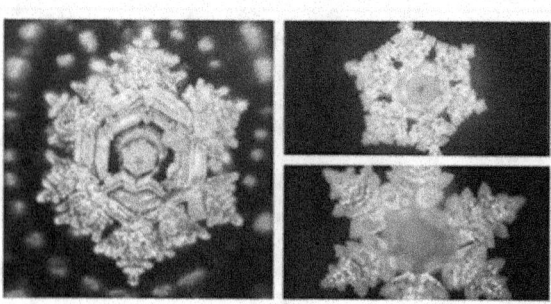

You are applying this science to make manifest Your POWER!

Its already IN YOU ….. with this book, you will create the Words for Your Own Story of Healing, Health, Life, Power and Greatness!!!

If a person is positive, cheerful and optimistic, it can change how other persons around him or she will feel. That person can, just by being close to others, spread positive energy.

There are many real-life proofs that being positive (just like negativity) spreads and it's the same with positive and negative words (words of gratitude, affection, complimenting words), music and songs that spread positivity, even nice pictures.

The water in us reacts to those positive things and because of that, we need to say positive words to ourselves on a constant and consistent basis. Your positive words will not only make you feel better, they will Shape You INTO them.

Understand that its not just the Word …. It's the Energy associated with the word.

Supreme Health & Fitness!   Knowledge Of Self Series Vol 2!

Affirm * Confirm * Claim Your Life!

As you Think, Write, Speak and Listen to Your story of Healing, Health, Life, Power and Greatness, you create Vibration at every stage. The Strength and Power of the Vibration is a result of the particular word used.

ALL WATER ABSORBS, REACTS IS AFFECTED BY VIBRATION!!!!

In this case, YOU or more specifically YOUR WORDS are the Cause of the Vibrations...... which means YOU ARE SHAPING YOURSELF INTO YOUR OWN SELF!!!!!!

YOU CAN CAUSE YOUR OWN HEALING!!!!

YOU CAN EMPOWER YOURSELF!!!!!

YOU CAN SUCCESSFULLY ENJOY YOUR ABUNDANT LIFE!!!!

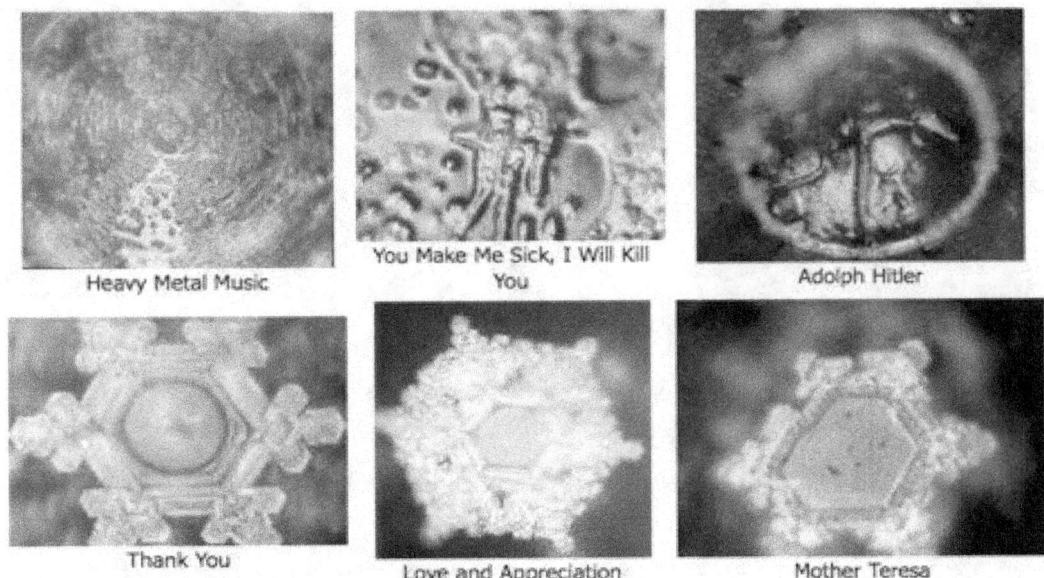

*Affirm * Confirm * Claim Your Life!*

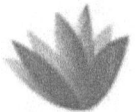 Gratitude Journal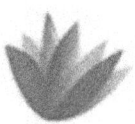

MORNING GRATITUDE PRAYER
Before you begin your day, list 10 things you're grateful for (big or small!).

1.
2.
3.
4.
5.
6.
7.
8.
9.
10.

WHAT I'M LEARNING FROM MY CHALLENGES
List 3 challenging situations, people, or other obstacles and what good thing you're learning from this challenge.

1.

I'm learning:

2.

I'm learning:

3.

I'm learning:

PEOPLE I'M THANKFUL FOR
List 5 people who made your life a little happier today. They could be friends, family, or even strangers!

1.
2.
3.
4.
5.

THE BEST PART OF MY DAY
Choose one moment of your day that made you happy and focus on it for 5 minutes before you go to sleep.

Affirm * Confirm * Claim Your Life!

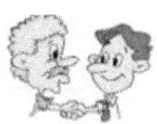 # RESPECT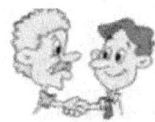

1. What is your definition of *RESPECT*?

2. What are some other words (synonyms) you may use for *RESPECT*?

3. Why is showing *RESPECT* so important?

4. Who should we *RESPECT*?

5. Who do you *RESPECT* the most in your life and why?

6. List 3 people you *RESPECT* and give examples how you could practically show *RESPECT*?

I *RESPECT* _____
and show *RESPECT* by…

I *RESPECT* _____
and show *RESPECT* by…

I *RESPECT* _____
and show *RESPECT* by…

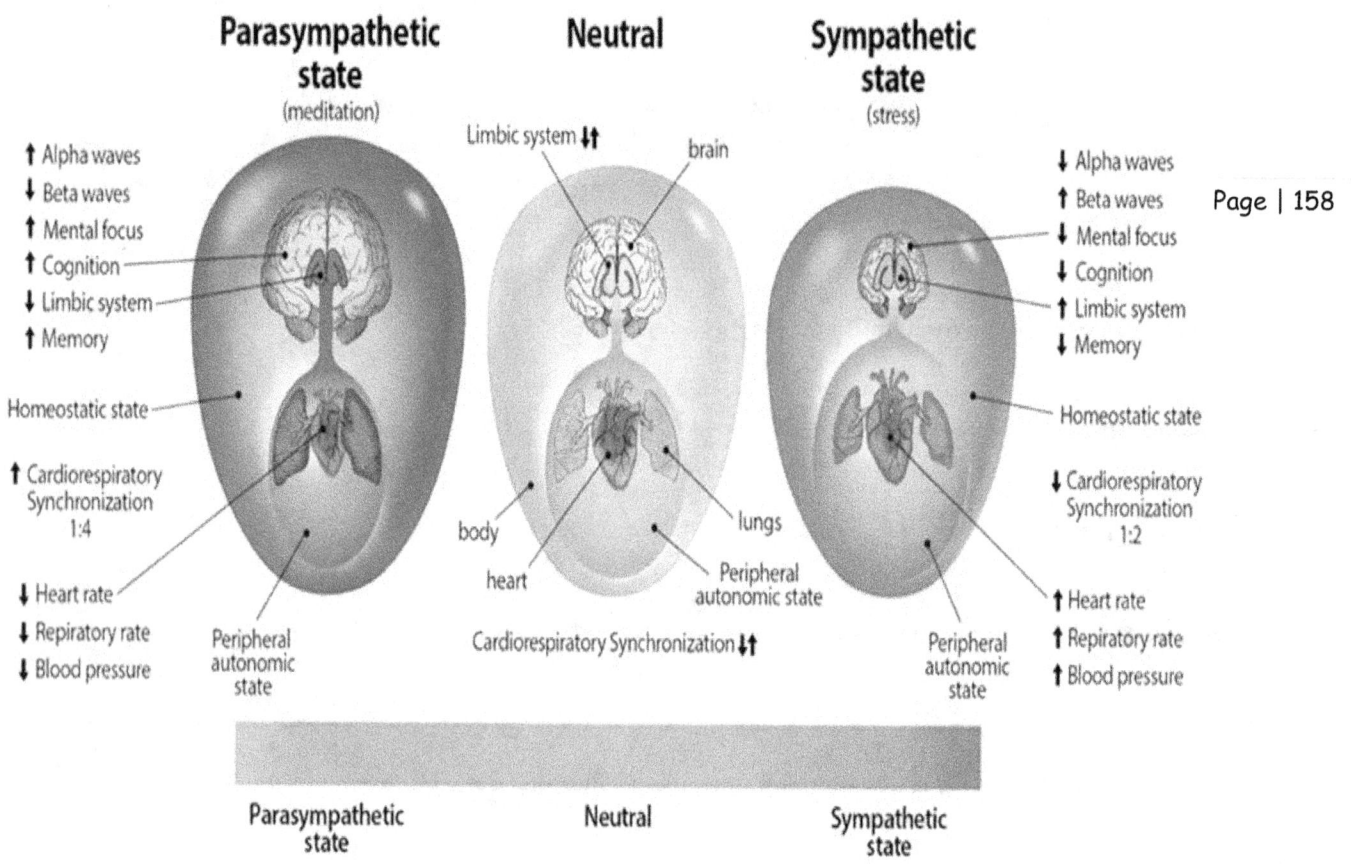

Representation of Mind-Body Response During Meditation and Stress

- I make time for me.
- I deserve to be well cared for.
- Self-nurture reminds me that I matter.
- I'm a good caregiver to myself.
- My physical, mental, and emotional well-being are a top priority.
- I take responsibility for my personal well-being.
- I take care of others by taking care of myself first.

*Affirm * Confirm * Claim Your Life!*

> The only reason you have not already received what you desire is because you are holding yourself in a vibrational pattern that does not match the vibration of your desire.

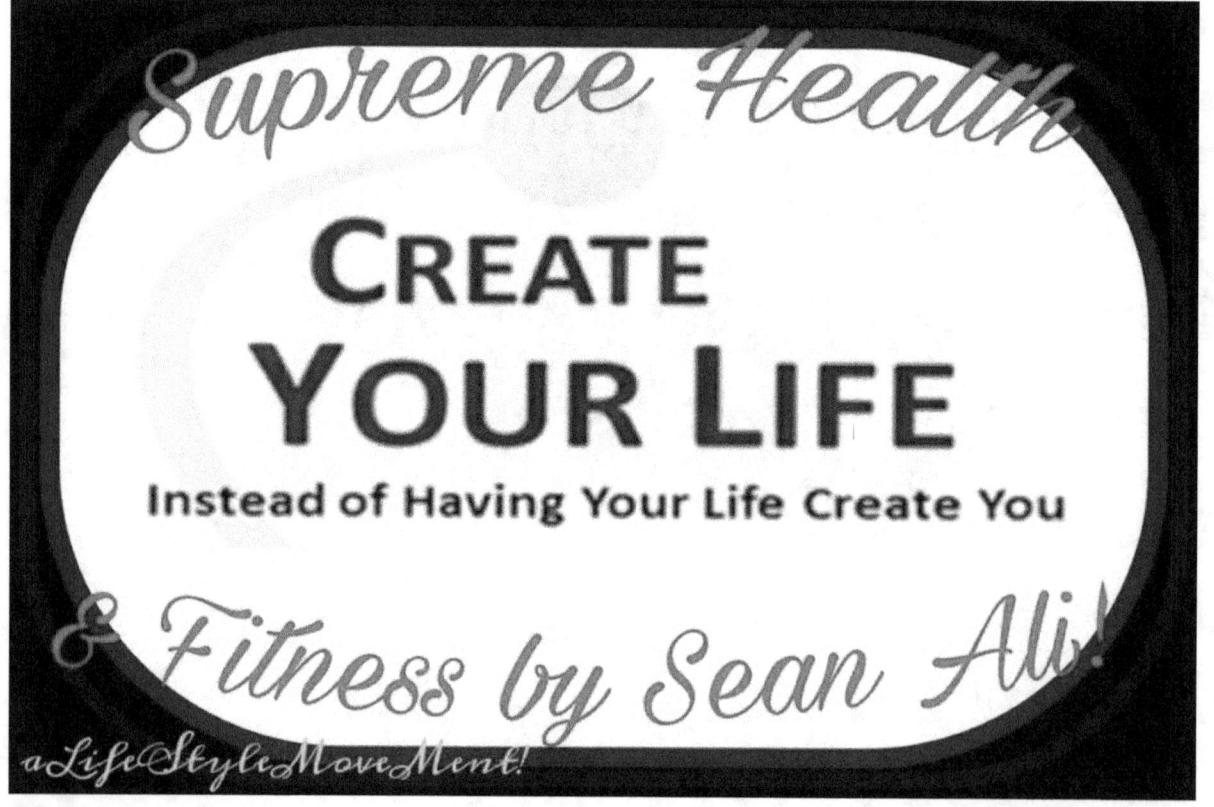

*Affirm * Confirm * Claim Your Life!*

Open To Create ...

EMOTIONAL INTELLIGENCE: Personal Review

> "Anyone can be angry - that is easy. But to be angry with the right person, to the right degrees at the right time, for the right purpose, and in the right way—that is not easy." - **Aristotle**

Exercise: Consider the questions below and score yourself out of ten for each one (ten being high). Consider your responses and notice areas where you scored 'low'. These are your areas for potential growth and may also indicate your personal vulnerabilities and greatest challenges. Also, notice where you confidently scored 'high' - these areas have the potential to support your challenges.

Emotional Intelligence	Score 10	Notes to self
Emotional Management		
If you are sad, grieving or mourning, do you allow yourself to cry? Can you cry openly in front of others?		
Can you express anger freely and non-destructively and then let it go?		
Do you quickly let go of grudges and resentment?		
When you are afraid, do you let trusted others see your fear?		
Are you able to recognise when you need help, then ask for help or support?		
Can you receive help, as well as give it?		
Can you say 'no' without feeling guilty?		
Can you strongly protest against mistreatment of self or others?		
Do you easily express, as well as receive, tenderness, love, passion?		
Can you enjoy your own company yet gladly and comfortably accept intimacy?		
Do you listen clearly to yourself and to others?		
Can you empathise with the needs and feelings of others, without judgement or criticism?		
Can you motivate others without resorting to fear tactics or manipulation?		
Do you allow yourself to frequently experience and enjoy pleasure?		

*Affirm * Confirm * Claim Your Life!*

Open To Create...

When necessary, can you contain (rather than repress), your impulses and delay your gratification, without resorting to guilt, shame, or suppression of your emotions?		
Do you allow yourself to experience bliss, ecstasy, excitement, fascination and awe?		
Do you often laugh out loud — a deep belly laugh?		
Do you sometimes feel moved by the courage or the spirit of others?		
Flexibility and balance		
Can you focus your energy on work, yet balance this with fun and rest?		
Can you accept and even enjoy others who have different needs and world-views?		
Do you let yourself be spontaneous, play like a child, be silly?		
Are your goals realistic, and does your patience allow you to work towards them steadily?		
Self awareness and positive esteem		
Can you forgive yourself your mistakes, and take yourself lightly?		
Can you accept your own shortcomings, without feeling ashamed, and remain excited about learning and growing?		
Do you respect your strengths and vulnerabilities, rather than inflate with pride, or fester with shame?		
Would you say you are generally true to yourself without blindly rebelling against, nor conforming to social expectations?		
Can you bear disappointment or frustration, without succumbing to criticism of self or others?		
Are you kind to yourself, do you avoid being hard — even punishing towards yourself?		

*Affirm * Confirm * Claim Your Life!*

Chapter Nine

Developing Your Creativity!

. . . . .

With this Chapter, You will examine and use the these 5 Basic Principles and Components to develop and build Your Creative Thinking Skills!

You will use Your Creative Skills to Re-Define YourSelf!

You will use Your Create Skills to produce the Vision for Your Healing!

You will use Your Creative Skills to make Manifest Your POWER!!!!!

Creative Thinking skills

Let's start with the following premise:

You're alive,

Therefore you're creative.

1. *Expertise*—a well-developed base of knowledge—furnishes the ideas, images, and phrases we use as mental building blocks. "Chance favors only the prepared mind," observed Louis Pasteur. The more blocks we have, the more chances we have to combine them in novel ways.

2. *Imaginative thinking skills* provide the ability to see things in novel ways, to recognize patterns, and to make connections. Having mastered a problem's basic elements, we redefine or explore it in a new way. Copernicus first developed expertise regarding the solar system and its planets, and then creatively defined the system as revolving around the Sun, not the Earth. Wiles' imaginative solution combined two partial solutions.

3. ***A venturesome personality*** seeks new experiences, tolerates ambiguity and risk, and perseveres in overcoming obstacles. Wiles said he labored in near-isolation from the mathematics community partly to stay focused and avoid distraction.

Such determination is an enduring trait.

4. ***Intrinsic motivation*** is being driven more by interest, satisfaction, and challenge than by external pressures (Amabile & Hennessey, 1992). Creative people focus less on extrinsic motivators—meeting deadlines, impressing people, or making money—than on the pleasure and stimulation of the work itself. Asked how he solved such difficult scientific problems, Isaac Newton reportedly answered, "By thinking about them all the time."

5. ***A creative environment*** sparks, supports, and refines creative ideas. Wiles stood on the shoulders of others and collaborated with a former student. After studying the careers of 2026 prominent scientists and inventors, Dean Keith Simonton (1992) noted that the most eminent were mentored, challenged, and supported by their colleagues. Creativity-fostering environments support innovation, team building, and communication (Hülsheger et al., 2009). They also support contemplation.

Whole Brain Creativity

ANALYTICAL
- Defines the problem by developing a clear picture of the current situation
- Has ideas focused on refining
- Selects solutions based on pros/cons analysis
- Emphasizes metrics

CONCEPTUAL
- Defines the problem by comparing to a clear vision for the future
- Has novel, transformational ideas
- Gets things started, tends to lose energy at implementation
- Paints a picture

STRUCTURAL
- Focuses on process and procedure
- Ideas focus on improving efficiency and effectiveness while retaining structure
- Is energized by plans, initiatives and implementation
- Seeks closure

SOCIAL
- Brings people together to discuss and define the problem
- Is attracted to problems involving interpersonal interaction
- Looks to see what others are doing (best practices)
- Motivates and encourages

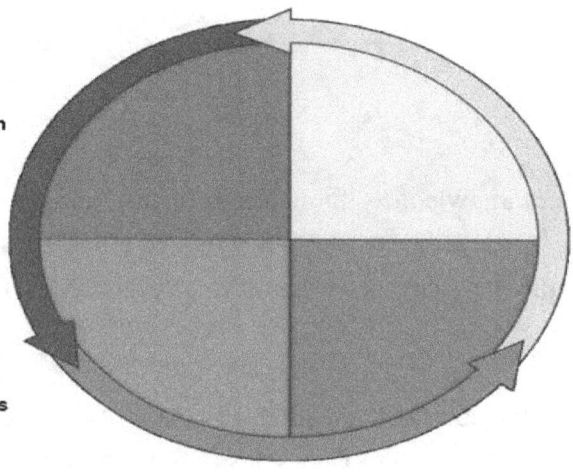

Fostering Your Own Creativity

Creative achievement springs from creativity-spawning persons and situations. To grow your own creativity,

- *develop your expertise.* Ask yourself what you care about and most enjoy. Follow your passion and become an expert at something.

- *allow time for incubation.* Given sufficient knowledge available for novel connections, a period of inattention to a problem ("sleeping on it") allows for unconscious processing to form associations (Zhong et al., 2008). So, think hard on a problem, then set it aside and come back to it later.

- *set aside time for the mind to roam freely.* Take time away from attention-absorbing television, social networking, and video gaming. Jog, go for a long walk, or meditate.

- *experience other cultures and ways of thinking.* Living abroad sets the creative juices flowing. Even after controlling for other variables, students who have spent time abroad are more adept at working out creative solutions to problems (Leung et al., 2008; Maddux et al., 2009, 2010). Multicultural experiences expose us to multiple perspectives and facilitate flexible thinking.

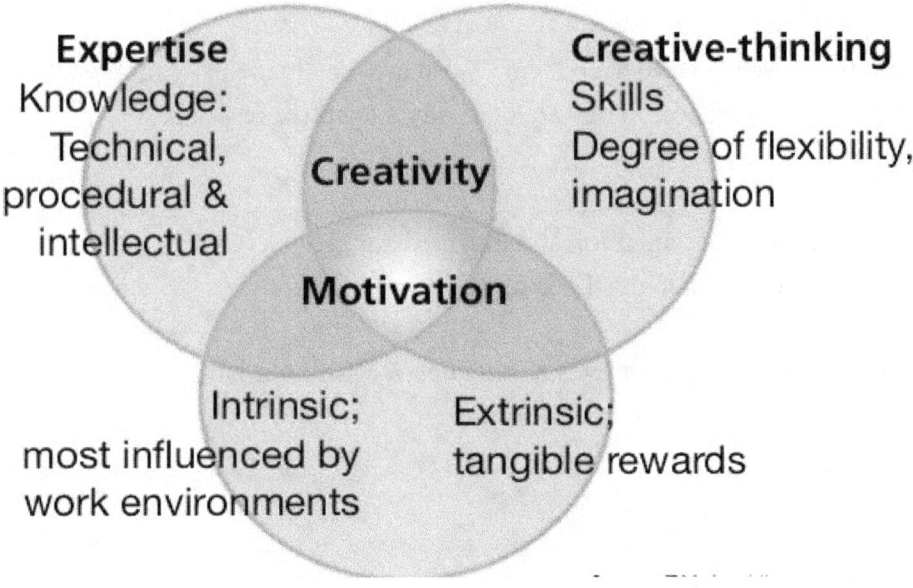

Discipline also refines talent. By their early twenties, top violinists have accumulated some 10,000 lifetime practice hours—double the practice time of other violin students aiming to be teachers (Ericsson 2001, 2006, 2007). From his studies, Herbert Simon (1998), a psychologist who won a Nobel Prize in Economics, formed what's called the *10-year rule:*

World-class experts in a field typically have invested "at least 10 years of hard work—say, 40 hours a week for 50 weeks a year." A study of outstanding scholars, athletes, and artists found that all were highly motivated and self-disciplined, willing to dedicate hours every day to the pursuit of their goals (Bloom, 1985). These superstar achievers were distinguished not so much by their extraordinary natural talent as by their extraordinary daily discipline.

What distinguishes extremely successful individuals from their equally talented peers, note Duckworth and Seligman, is *grit*—passionate dedication to an ambitious, long-term goal. Although intelligence is distributed like a bell curve, achievements are not.

That tells us that achievement involves much more than raw ability. That is why organizational psychologists seek ways to engage and motivate ordinary people doing ordinary jobs. And that is why training students in "hardiness"—resilience under stress—leads to better grades (Maddi et al., 2009).

How do arousal, cognition, and expressive behavior interact in emotion?

Motivated behavior is often connected to powerful emotions

Where do such emotions come from? Why do we have them? What are they made of? Emotions don't exist just to give us interesting experiences. They are our body's adaptive response, increasing our chances of survival.

When we face challenges, emotions focus our attention and energize our actions (Cyders & Smith, 2008). Our heart races. Our pace quickens. All our senses go on high alert.

Receiving unexpected good news, we may find our eyes tearing up. We raise our hands triumphantly. We feel exuberance and a newfound confidence.

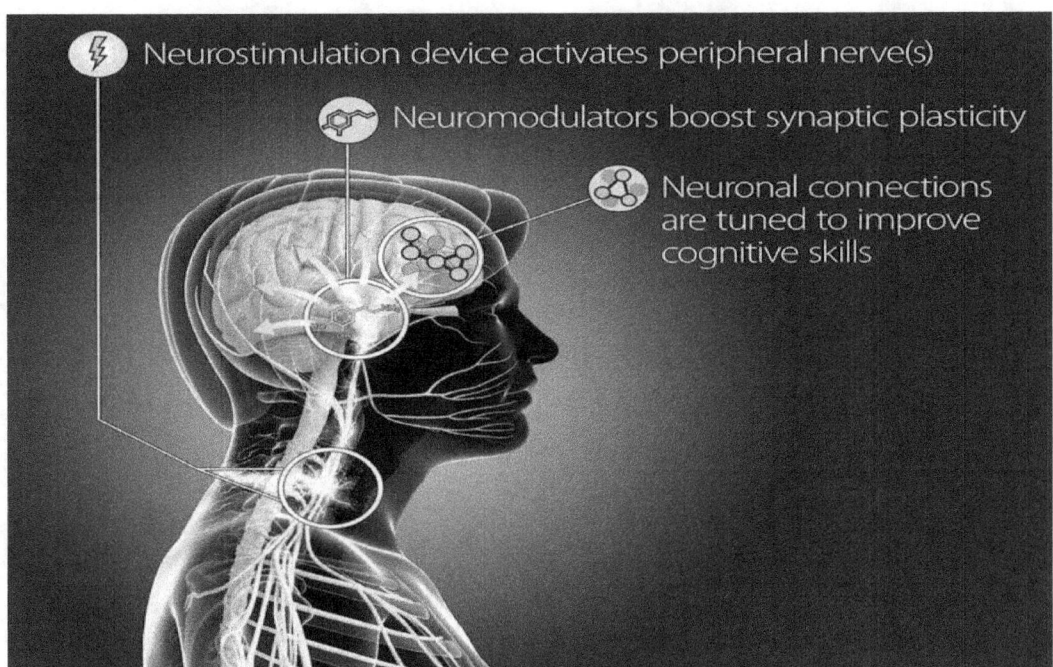

Creative vs Critical thinking

Creative thinking is described as:
- making and communicating connections to think of many possibilities;
- think and experience in various ways and use different points of view;
- think of new and unusual possibilities; and
- guide in generating and selecting alternatives.

Critical thinking is described as:
- analyzing and developing possibilities to compare and contrast many ideas
- improve and refine ideas
- make effective decisions and judgments, and
- provide a sound foundation for effective action.

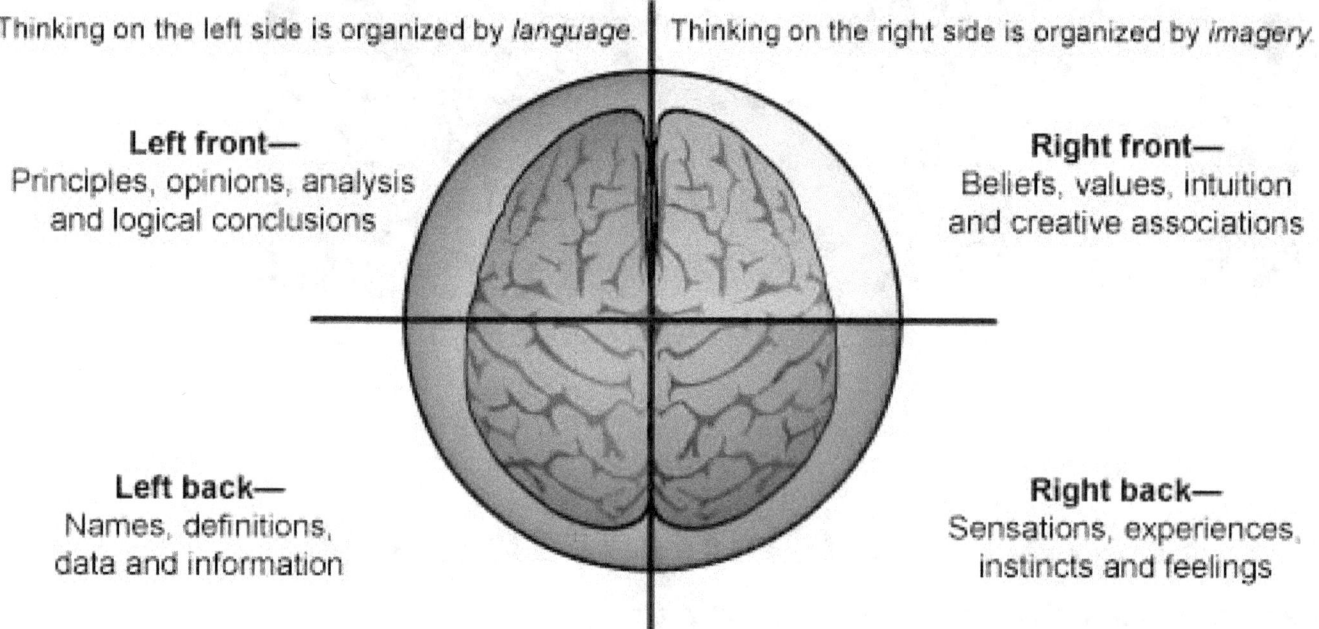

Affirm * Confirm * Claim Your Life!

Chapter Ten

Guidelines – Improving Perception

* * * * *

The main focus on improving our Perception and Communication skills is so they we can properly Perceive OURSELVES and effectively Communicate with OURSELVES!

This is where our Healing, Health, Life and Power is manifested and cultivated from. We have to Improve HOW we SEE ourselves and HOW we TALK to and about ourselves. We use and Improved Perception about ourselves to Successfully RE-Define ourselves according to our own Definitions and Create ourselves as we want.

Improved Communication is HOW we WILL into Existence our Thoughts and Ideas!

We are God's, Created IN the Image and Likeness of GOD! All God has to DO is SAY BE – and It IS!

This is Communication!

We are striving to build up our Energy to Will (Say/Communicate) into existence our Healing, Health, Life and Power!

Many of us cannot do this for ourselves now …. Because this requires Improved Communication within ourselves.

Because perception is a foundation of interpersonal communication, it's important to form perceptions carefully and check their accuracy. Here, we discuss seven guidelines for improving the accuracy of perceptions and, ultimately, the quality of interpersonal communication.

Affirm * Confirm * Claim Your Life!

Recognize That All Perceptions Are Partial and Subjective

Our perceptions are always partial and subjective. They are partial because we cannot perceive everything; and they are subjective because they are influenced by factors such as culture, physiology, roles, standpoint, and cognitive abilities.

Objective features of reality have no meaning until we notice, organize, and interpret them. It is our perceptions that construct meanings for the people and experiences in our lives. Each of us perceives from a particular perspective that is shaped by our physiology, culture, standpoint, social roles, cognitive abilities, and personal experiences. An outfit perceived as elegant by one person may appear cheap to another.

The **subjective** and **partial** nature of perceptions has implications for interpersonal communication. One implication is that, when you and another person disagree about something, neither of you is necessarily wrong. It's more likely that you have attended to different things and that there are differences in your personal, social, cultural, cognitive, and physiological resources for perceiving.

A second implication is that it's wise to remind ourselves that our perceptions are based at least as much on ourselves as on anything external to us.

Remembering that perceptions are partial and subjective curbs the tendency to think that our perceptions are the only valid ones or that they are based exclusively on what lies outside us.

Check Perceptions

Because perceptions are subjective and partial, and because mind reading is an ineffective way to figure out what others think, we need to check our perceptions with others.

Perception checking is an important communication skill because it helps people arrive at mutual understandings of each other and their relationships. To check perceptions, you should first state what you have noticed.

Distinguish between Facts and Inferences

Competent interpersonal communication also depends on distinguishing facts from inferences. A fact is based on observation. An inference involves an interpretation that goes beyond the facts.

For example, suppose that you are consistently late reporting to work and sometimes dozes off during discussions. Coworkers might think, "You person is lazy and unmotivated." The facts are that you come in late and sometimes falls asleep. Defining You as lazy and unmotivated is an inference that goes beyond the facts.

More often than not we do the same above scenario WITH OURSELVES. We can easily take our own weaknesses or short-comings and infer on ourselves that because we are late or tired that we are lazy, when the FACT is that we were just late and tired.

But just as the outside Inference can mislead, when we do it to ourselves, it creates the negative and destructive environment of self-doubt, self-loathing and the inability to see the Quality and Greatness of ourselves.

Guard against the Fundamental Attribution Error

We've also discussed a second error in interpretation: the fundamental attribution error. This occurs when we overestimate the internal causes of others' undesirable behavior and underestimate the external causes, and when we underestimate the internal causes of our own failings or bad behaviors and overestimate the external causes. We need to guard against this error because it distorts our perceptions of ourselves and others.

Instead of letting yourself off the hook by explaining a misdeed as caused by circumstances you couldn't control, ask yourself, "What factor inside of me that is my responsibility influenced what I did?" Looking for external factors that influence others' communication and internal factors that influence your own communication checks our tendency to make fundamental attribution errors.

Monitor Labels

In giving names to our perceptions, we clarify them to ourselves. But just as words crystallize experiences, they can also freeze thought. **Once we label our perceptions, we may respond to our own labels rather than to actual phenomena. If this happens, we may communicate in insensitive and inappropriate ways.**

When we engage in interpersonal communication, we abstract only certain aspects of the total reality around us. Our perceptions are one step away from reality because they are always partial and subjective. We move a second step from reality when we label a perception. We move even farther from the actual reality when we respond not to behaviors or our perceptions of them but instead to the label we impose. This process can be illustrated as a ladder of abstraction a concept emphasized by one of the first scholars of interpersonal communication (Hayakawa, 1962, 1964).

We should also monitor our labels to adapt our communication to particular people. Competent interpersonal communicators are sensitive to others and their preferences and choose their words accordingly. This is especially important when we are talking with or about identities.

Perceiving accurately is neither magic nor an ability that some people naturally possess. Instead, it is a communication skill that can be developed and practiced. Following the seven guidelines we have discussed will allow you to perceive more carefully and more accurately in interpersonal communication.

*Affirm * Confirm * Claim Your Life!*

THE ULTIMATE guide to Self-Compassion

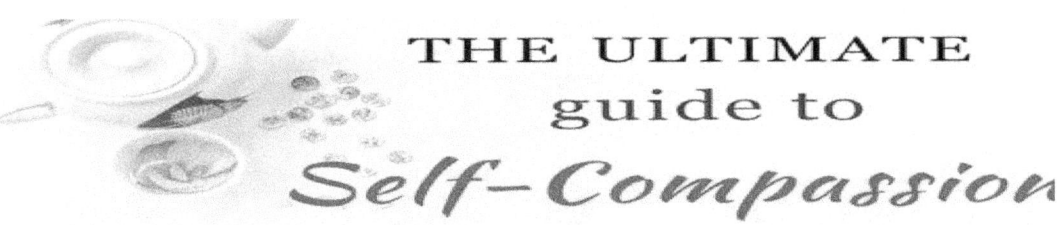

Three Elements of Self-compassion

1. Self-kindness
"What I'm going through is very hard right now."

2. Common Humanity
"What I'm going through is hard, but I'm not alone. Everybody goes through adversity."

3. Mindfulness
"I am here and I see you."

Self-compassion IS NOT: 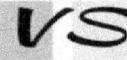 Self-compassion IS:

IS NOT:
- Selfishness & Narcissism
- Judgment & Criticism
- Self-pity
- Self-indulgence

IS:
- Self-compassion quiets down the ego and minimizes the egoistic sense of self without ignoring or suppressing the self's needs
- Having a kind understanding and an open mind, and acceptance.
- Self-compassion allows us to step back and take the approach of other towards oneself.
- Caring awareness which allows us to listen to our bodies and find out what is healthy for us.

Benefits of Self-compassion

- Motivation and self-improvement
- Eudaimonic happiness
- Lowered symptoms of depression

How to put self-compassion into practice

- Cultivate mindfulness
- Hug yourself and speak to yourself softly
- Practice loving kindness meditation
- Cultivate forgiveness towards self
- Write a letter to yourself from a perspective of unconditional acceptance

Affirm * Confirm * Claim Your Life!

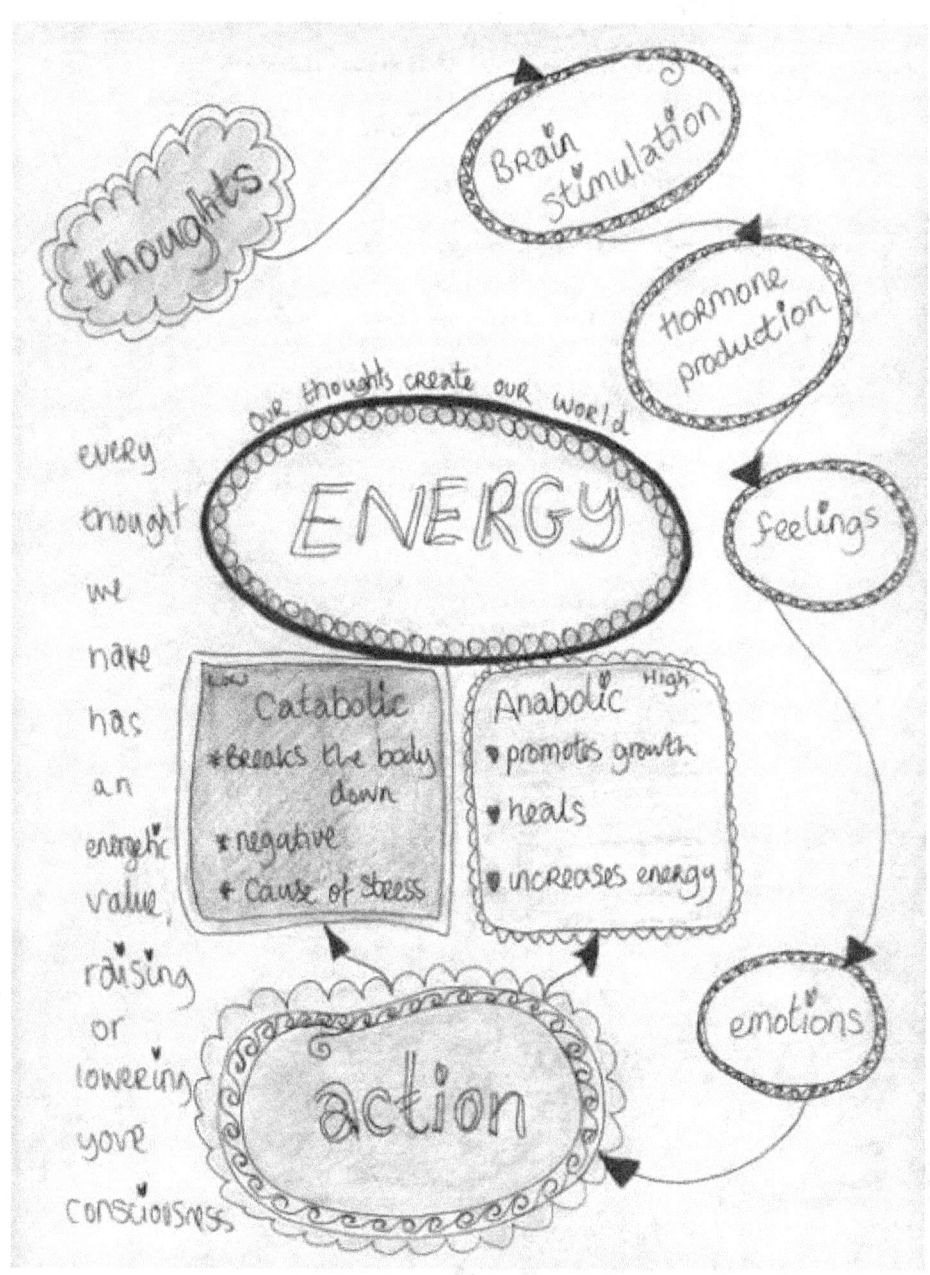

*Affirm * Confirm * Claim Your Life!*

Personal Development Action Plan

In order to reach your goals what behaviours will you STOP, MINIMISE, KEEP DOING, do MORE of and which will you START?

	STOP	MINIMISE	KEEP DOING	Do MORE	START
1					
2					
3					
4					
5					

SKILLS TO USE TO REGULATE EMOTIONS

#	(A) CORE SKILLS	(B) DISTRACTION	(C) SELF-SOOTHE
1	DEEP BREATHING	COUNT NUMBERS	TAKE A LONG BATH
2	OBSERVE & DESCRIBE	WATCH TV	DRINK DECAF TEA
3	RADICAL ACCEPTANCE	COLOR/PAINT/DRAW	LIGHT CANDLES
4	MINDFULNESS/AWARENESS	WORK A PUZZLE	LISTEN TO SOOTHING MUSIC
5	HELP SOMEONE ELSE	EXERCISE	POSITIVE SELF-AFFIRMATIONS
6	PROS & CONS LIST	CALL A FRIEND	USE COMFORT BOX
7	PUSH AWAY THOUGHTS	CALL YOUR SPONSOR	TAKE A "VACATION"

I was born to achieve
I create my own destiny
All the resources I will ever need are within me

I will love and respect myself every day of my life

It's not what happens in life, it's my reaction to what happens

Champions are people like me
My positive thoughts lead to positive actions
Problems are opportunities that make me stronger

Treating people with respect will assure my future

Leaders are learners

*Affirm * Confirm * Claim Your Life!*

Claim!

* * * * *

This is the ACTION stage!!

This is where you put into ACTION all the Healing and Powerful Affirm and Confirm statements!

A change in behavior does not happen without practice. The metacognitive term is rehearse, a robust form of practice.

Rehearse involves studying the situation, preparing to meet expectations, running through the actual sequence of completing the assigned task or test, and then repeating the actions for the purpose of improving your performance or outcome.

The rehearse phase allows your Patterns to go through a trial run to make certain that the performance of the task, the completion of the project, and/or the public presentation will meet the standards set by the instructor.

Rehearsal prepares for expression by allowing any mistakes to be identified and corrected in advance of submitting the final product.

You begin the Claim process by Writing your Claim statements, wherein you place Claim on your previous Affirm and Confirm statements.

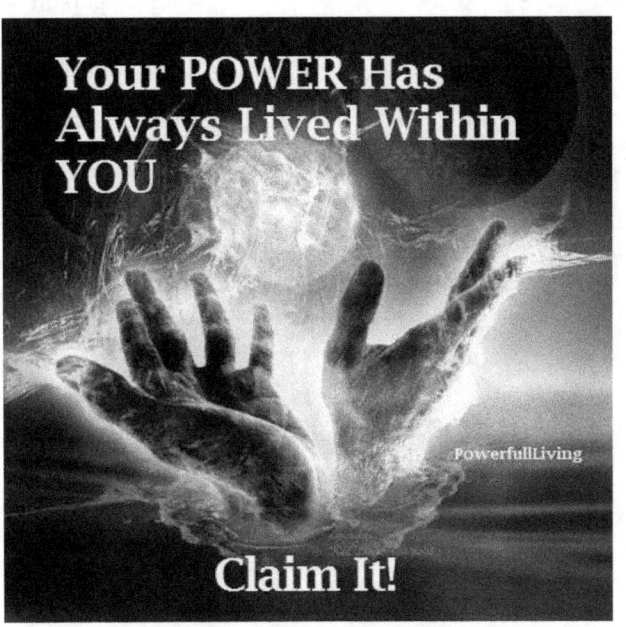

Affirm * Confirm * Claim Your Life!

Example: I CLAIM My Health!   I CLAIM My Power!   I CLAIM My Life!
I CLAIM My Intelligence!

After you Write your Claim statements, you now have a PERFECT Blueprint to CLAIM YOUR HEALING, HEALTH, LIFE AND POWER!!!!

You have Successfully written Your Own story of Healing!

You have Successfully written Your Own story of Health!

You have Successfully written Your Own story of Life!

You have Successfully written Your Own story of Power!

Now all You have to DO is Walk right INTO Your Story!!!

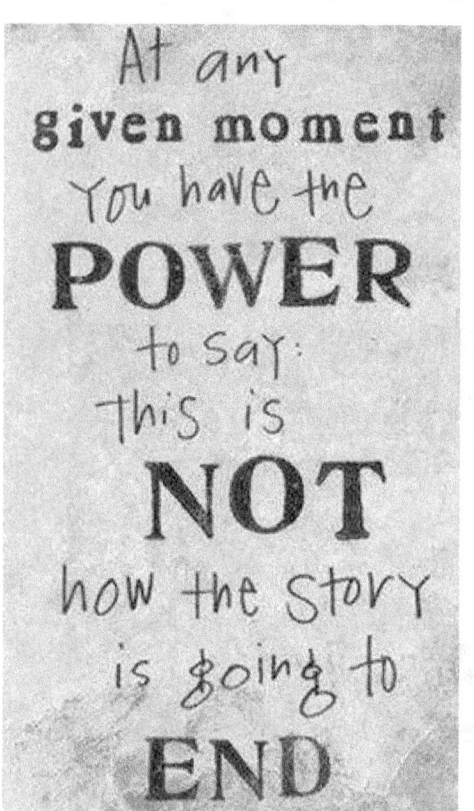

As you travel and need Motivation, all you have to do is OPEN Your Own Book and get Motivated from Your Own story!

The foundation of this WorkBook is designed to place your ability to find Encourage and the ability to Succeed from YOURSELF. so instead of having to find Inspiration from another person's story, YOU CAN GET IT FROM YOUR OWN!!!!

That is placing your Power IN YOU!

Affirm * Confirm * Claim Your Life!

I CLAIM My _____!

I CLAIM My _____!

I CLAIM My _____!

I CLAIM My _____!

I CLAIM My _____!

I CLAIM My _____!

I CLAIM My _____!

I CLAIM My _____!

I CLAIM My _____!

I CLAIM My _____!

I CLAIM My _____!

I CLAIM My _____!

I CLAIM My _____!

I CLAIM My _____!

I CLAIM My _____!

I CLAIM My _____!

I CLAIM My _____!

I CLAIM My _____!

Affirm * Confirm * Claim Your Life!

I CLAIM My _____!

I CLAIM My _____!

I CLAIM My _____!

I CLAIM My _____!

I CLAIM My _____!

I CLAIM My _____!

I CLAIM My _____!

I CLAIM My _____!

I CLAIM My _____!

I CLAIM My _____!

I CLAIM My _____!

I CLAIM My _____!

I CLAIM My _____!

I CLAIM My _____!

I CLAIM My _____!

I CLAIM My _____!

I CLAIM My _____!

I CLAIM My _____!

*Affirm * Confirm * Claim Your Life!*

5 Daily Reminders

1. I am amazing.
2. I can do anything.
3. Positivity is a choice.
4. I celebrate my individuality.
5. I am prepared to succeed.

Reflective Practice—Assess, Reflect, Revisit

The final phases of metacognition form the basis of something called reflective practice, which is actually a part of critical thinking. Reflective practice is also known as double-looped learning because it takes you back to examine the defining questions you asked yourself as you entered into doing the assignment (your assumptions, actions, and decisions) and the results you achieved at the conclusion (success, partial success, or failure). Reflective practice allows you to learn from your decisions and actions while determining their effectiveness. Don't skip these vital stages, as they help you gain confidence and avoid repeating any mistakes.

Affirm * Confirm * Claim Your Life!

Assess

The metacognitive phases, when faithfully followed, always include a time to assess. Unlike external assessment or testing, the assess phase of metacognition means confronting questions internally, such as "What have I really achieved?" and "To what degree have I achieved it?"

You need to ask yourself, "What is the outcome of my effort?" and let the feedback from your instructor lead you to consider the results of your efforts. The metacognitive phase that follows links to this one—it too focuses on the question, "What is the outcome of my effort?"

Reflect

When you reflect, you begin your internal conversation with "As a result of my effort, I. . .." and you conclude with, "Next time, I will. . ." When you reflect, you ask, "Where does the buck stop? Who is responsible for this success? This failure? This mess?"

This is the piece of professional and personal growth you may have been missing. After all, anyone can use the phrase "mistakes have been made" to anonymously attribute failure and blame.

But only mindful individuals with a clear sense of their personal Learning Patterns face themselves (Osterman & Kottkamp, 2004) and say precisely, "I screwed up, and I am prepared to take the heat for it."

Nia, the Strong-Willed learner, avoids this phase of learning at all costs. Her unwillingness to reflect costs her. Using your metacognition well equips you to reach a powerful self-awareness and to be open to ask, "What did I allow myself to do? What did I fail to do? Where did my Learning Patterns steer me off course?"

This is the autopsy of failure and of success. Without intentionally focusing on your actions, approaches, and thoughts, you are doomed to continue to achieve less than you could. You cannot continue to repeat the same actions, believing that they will yield a different outcome.

*Affirm * Confirm * Claim Your Life!*

Reflection requires us to face ourselves—specifically how we have used our metacognitive talk and our self-correcting opportunities and how we have failed to do so. This is the key to being an intentional learner.

Revisit

The good news found in reflective practice is that it does not conclude with simply assigning blame or with rewarding success. Reflective practice invites you instead to revisit your metacognitive phases, noting both those that enriched and those that frustrated your venture. Revisiting metacognitive decisions serves to reinforce the specific strategies that led to success and to reconsider those that led to failure. Revisiting grows both metacognitive capacity and personal insight.

There is no doubt that when you understand your Learning Patterns and are aware of the internal talk of your Patterns as they work through the metacognitive phases, you are well equipped, as Peter Senge, the guru of professional development, describes, "to consistently enhance your capacity to produce results that are truly important to you" (1999, p. 45).

Reflection and Reflective Practice

Approaches to Learning

Surface Learning	Deep Learning
Intention to complete the task and memorize information.	Intention to understand and seek meaning.
	Attempt to relate concepts to existing experience.
No distinction between new ideas and existing knowledge.	Distinguish between new ideas and existing knowledge
	Critical evaluation of events.
Facts learned out with a meaningful framework.	Facts learned in the context of meaning.
Knowledge	**Understanding**

Affirm * Confirm * Claim Your Life!

Directions: Each of the following items asks you about your emotions or reactions associated with emotions. After deciding whether a statement is generally true for you, use the 5-point scale to respond to the statement. Please circle the "1" if you strongly disagree that this is like you, the "2" if you somewhat disagree that this is like you, "3" if you neither agree nor disagree that this is like you, the "4" if you somewhat agree that this is like you, and the "5" if you strongly agree that this is like you.

There are no right or wrong answers. Please give the response that best describes you.

1 = strongly disagree
2 = somewhat disagree
3 = neither agree nor disagree
4 = somewhat agree
5 = strongly agree

1. I know when to speak about my personal problems to others.   1   2   3   4   5
2. When I am faced with obstacles, I remember times I faced similar obstacles and overcame them.   1   2   3   4   5
3. I expect that I will do well on most things I try.   1   2   3   4   5
4. Other people find it easy to confide in me.   1   2   3   4   5
5. I find it hard to understand the non-verbal messages of other people.   1   2   3   4   5
6. Some of the major events of my life have led me to re-evaluate what is important and not important.   1   2   3   4   5
7. When my mood changes, I see new possibilities.   1   2   3   4   5
8. Emotions are one of the things that make my life worth living.   1   2   3   4   5
9. I am aware of my emotions as I experience them.   1   2   3   4   5
10. I expect good things to happen.   1   2   3   4   5
11. I like to share my emotions with others.   1   2   3   4   5
12. When I experience a positive emotion, I know how to make it last.   1   2   3   4   5
13. I arrange events others enjoy.   1   2   3   4   5
14. I seek out activities that make me happy.   1   2   3   4   5
15. I am aware of the non-verbal messages I send to others.   1   2   3   4   5

Affirm * Confirm * Claim Your Life!

MIND, BODY AND SPIRIT.

WEEKLY WELLNESS PLAN:

DATE: _____

TAKE CARE OF THE WHOLE YOU.
>>>>>>>

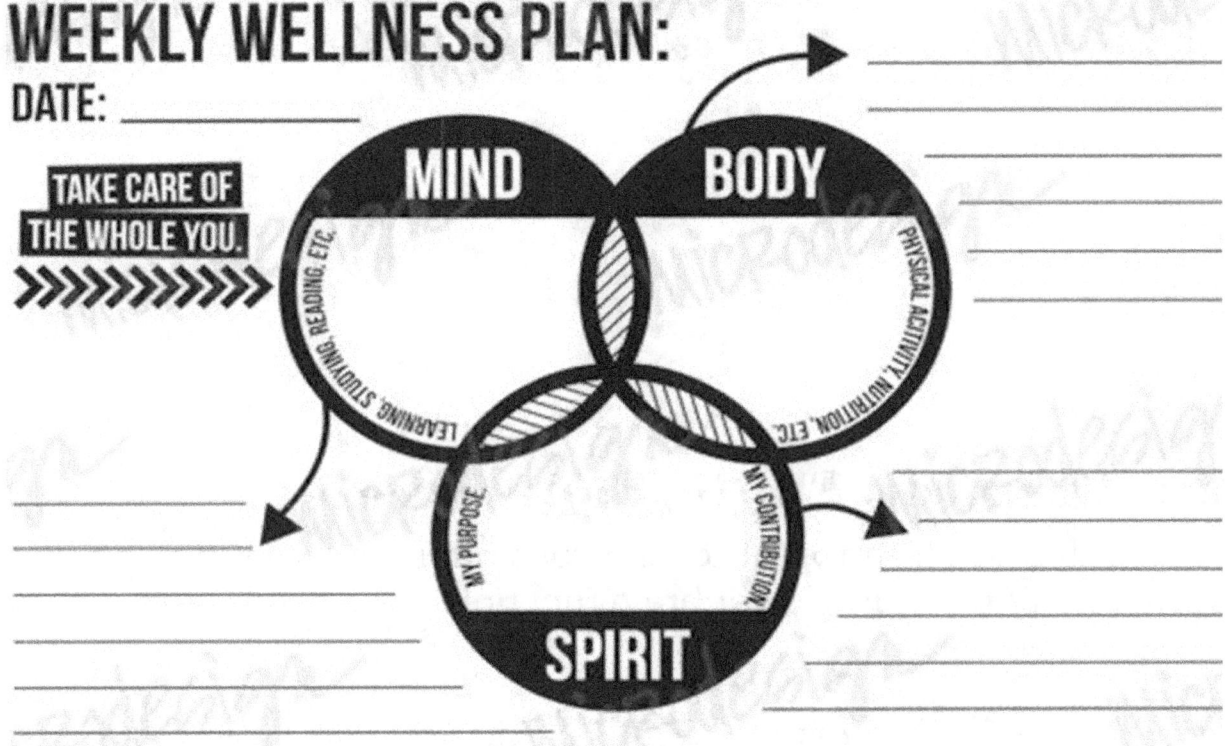

JOY KILLERS TO AVOID: ....

WEEKLY REFLECTIONS

WHAT WAS AWESOME ABOUT THIS WEEK? WHAT DO I WANT TO DO DIFFERENTLY NEXT WEEK?

*Affirm * Confirm * Claim Your Life!*

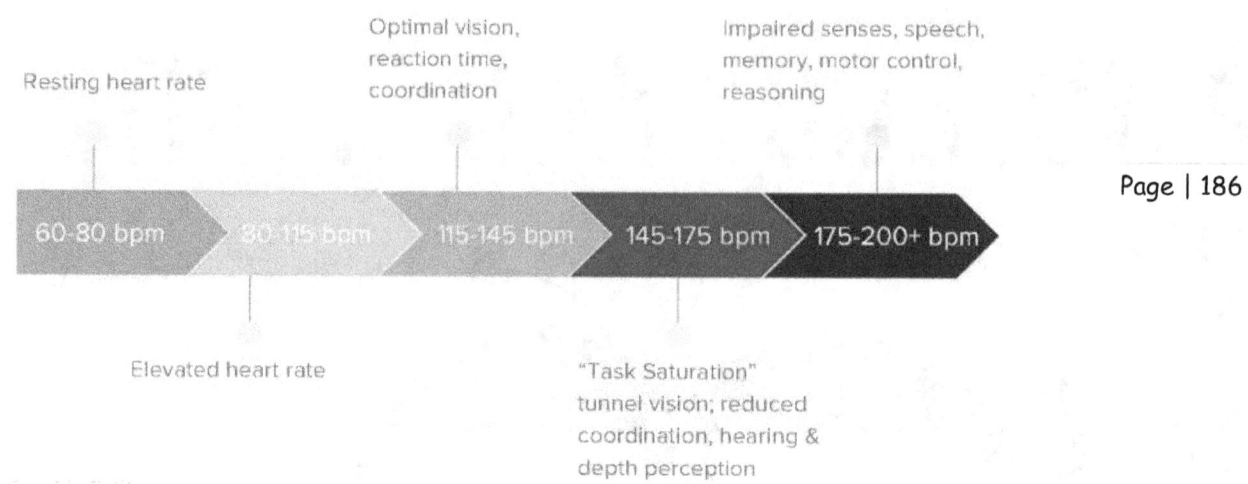

Survival Mode: Flight/Fight/Freeze
Frontal lobe (Prefrontal cortex) goes offline
Limbic system / mind and lower brain functions take over

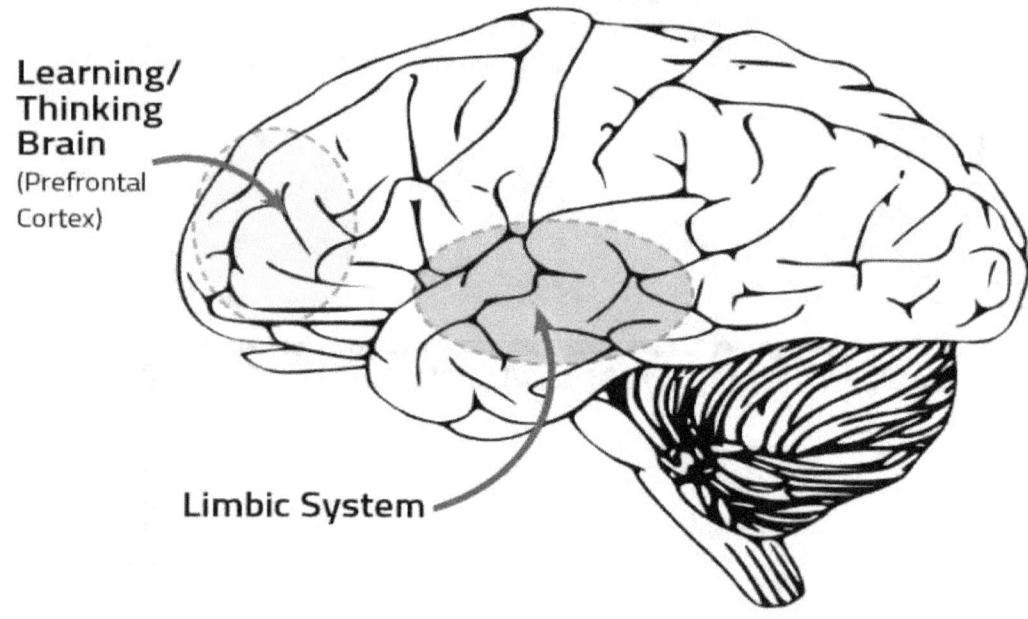

*Affirm * Confirm * Claim Your Life!*

Understanding FEAR!

* * * * *

FEAR is the one thing that prevents you from Re-Defining yourself and successfully creating the environment for Your Healing, Your Health, Your Life and Your Power!

FEAR OF THE UNKNOWN!

In this case FEAR represents – False Education Accepted as Reality

We have been falsely educated about ourselves and have accepted this false education as Reality.

We have lived the majority of our lives under the definitions placed on us from others. Many of us fear the unknown Self. We fear Claiming our own Power. We fear BEING the God's that we ARE!

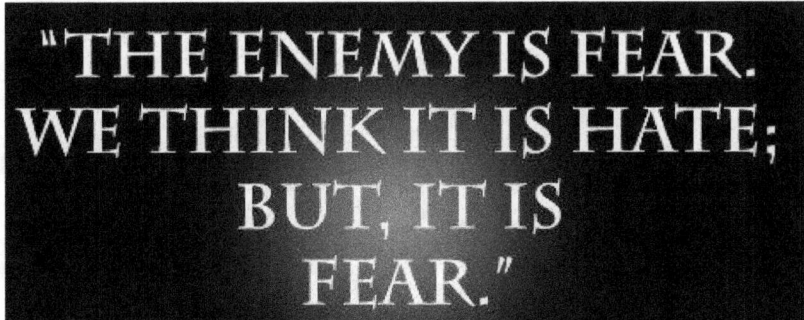

Why do we fear the wrong things? Psychologists have identified four influences that feed fear and cause us to ignore higher risks:

1. *We fear what our ancestral history has prepared us to fear.* Human emotions were road tested in the Stone Age. Our old brain prepares us to fear yesterday's risks: snakes, lizards, and spiders (which combined now kill a tiny fraction of the number killed by modern-day threats, such as cars and cigarettes). Yesterday's risks also prepare us to fear confinement and heights, and therefore flying.

2. *We fear what we cannot control.* Driving we control; flying we do not.

3. *We fear what is immediate.* The dangers of flying are mostly telescoped into the moments of takeoff and landing. The dangers of driving are diffused across many moments to come, each trivially dangerous.

4. *Thanks to the availability heuristic, we fear what is most readily available in memory.* Powerful, vivid images, like that of United Flight 175 slicing into the World Trade Center, feed our judgments of risk. Thousands of safe car trips have extinguished our anxieties about driving. Similarly, we remember (and fear) widespread disasters (hurricanes, tornadoes, earthquakes) that kill people dramatically, in bunches. But we fear too little the less dramatic threats that claim lives quietly, one by one, continuing into the distant future. Bill Gates has noted that each year a half-million children worldwide die from rotavirus. This is the equivalent of four 747s full of children every day, and we hear nothing of it (Glass, 2004).

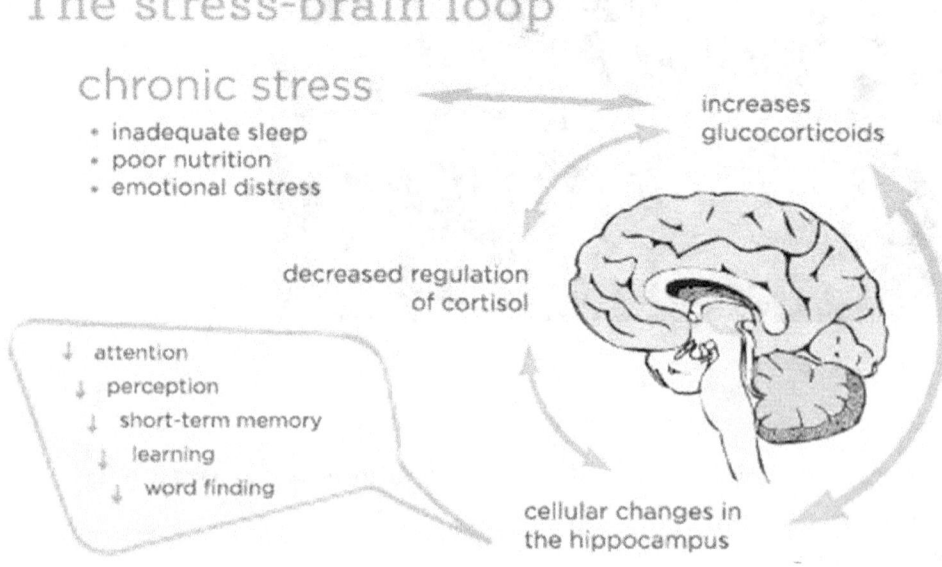

Affirm * Confirm * Claim Your Life!

**OUR DEEPEST FEAR
IS NOT THAT WE ARE INADEQUATE.
OUR DEEPEST FEAR
IS THAT WE ARE MORE
POWERFUL BEYOND MEASURE.
IT IS LIGHT,
NOT OUR DARKNESS THAT FRIGHTENS US.
WE ASK OURSELVES, WHO AM I TO BE BRILLIANT,
GORGEOUS, TALENTED, FABULOUS?
ACTUALLY, WHO ARE YOU NOT TO BE?**

Negative Message

Negative words and energies cause the crystals to be misshapen and ugly.

devil	I'll kill you	You fool	You crazy	You can't!	You die!
Before praying	Mystery circle	Raindrops	Separation	Heart Break	Yesterday

Sad music

Affirm * Confirm * Claim Your Life!

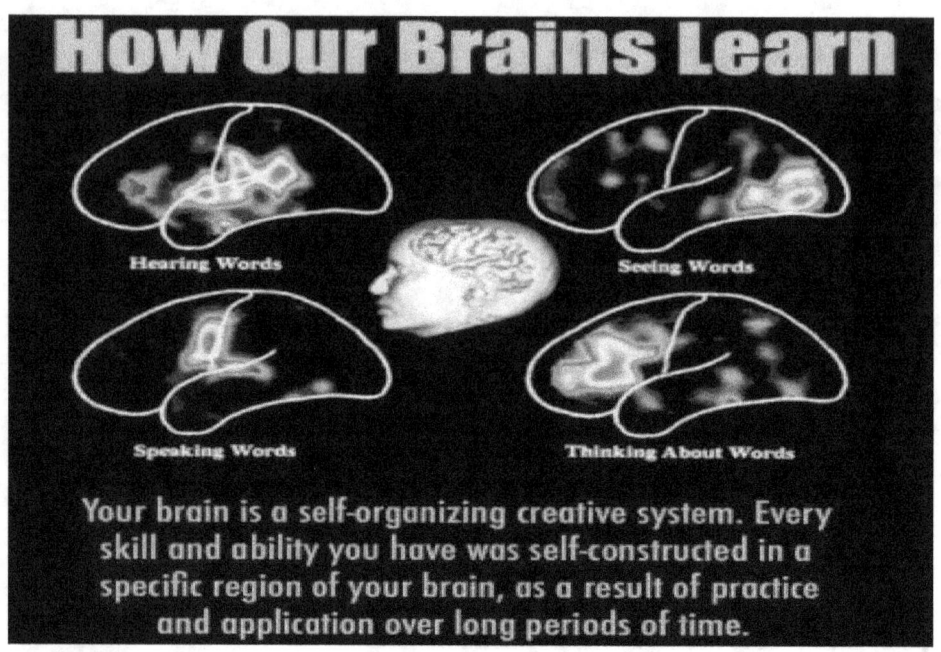

This is Your Chance to Build Your BRAIN according to How You WANT!!!

The Words You THINK about are Your HEALING, Your Life, Your Power and Your Greatness – Causing Your Brain to GROW into Your Words!

By Writing down these High Energy Power words, the Words that You SEE will Cause Your Brain to GROW into Your Words!!

By Speaking these Power Words – You Cause Your Brain to GROW into Your Words!!

By Hearing these Words of Your Healing, Life, Power and Greatness – You Cause Your Brain to GROW into Your Own Words!!

Your Brain is Your Control Center …. Where Your Brain or Thoughts go = Your Body Follows.

By Growing Your Brain INTO Your Healing – It Sends the corresponding Energy and Hormones to the rest of Your Body = GROWING Your Body INTO HEALING!!!!!

You Grow YOUR BODY INTO YOUR POWER!!!!!

You Grow YOUR BODY INTO YOUR GREATNESS!!!!

*Affirm * Confirm * Claim Your Life!*

"Develop your Emotional Intelligence!"

The following techniques and tips will enable you to progress at your own speed. They will provide you with food for thought for each of the test's eight themes, and help pave the way for your increased emotional independence.

Self-knowledge

A. Identify difficulties to better deal with them (fatigue, stress, anxiety, etc.)
B. Differentiate between good stress, which energizes, and bad stress, which drains
C. Get to know your limits and learn to set yourself reachable goals
D. Listen to others

Self-control

A. Learn to take it easy, to relax. Stress can be neutralized very simply
B. Learn to build moments of rest into your day, and to better organize yourself
C. A sane mind in a sane body: maintain a healthy life style, eat a balanced diet and don't neglect sports!
D. Tips for conquering stress (or stage fright)
E. Learn to analyze your anger and to get a better grip on it

*Affirm * Confirm * Claim Your Life!*

How to Build Confidence

Evaluate Your Confidence Levels

Statement	Strongly Agree	Agree	Neutral	Disagree	Strongly Disagree
I have a clear sense of what's important to me.					
I know what I want in life.					
I admit my mistakes and know that setbacks can be learned from.					
I can stand back and think clearly when things get emotional.					
Most of my work involves things I enjoy doing.					
I make other people feel good about themselves.					
People know me as being an optimistic.					
I respect myself and others.					
I am realistic about my strengths and weaknesses.					
I know what others consider to be my strengths.					
I freely ask for help.					
I am able to see the wider perspective and the smaller details of a situation.					
I enjoy taking on new challenges.					
I seek out opportunities to learn and grow.					
I take care of my mind and body.					
I handle stress with ease and don't take things too personally.					
I am clear about my purpose in life.					
I have positive yet realistic expectations.					
Even though I dive in to new opportunities I have a balanced perspective about risk taking.					

*Affirm * Confirm * Claim Your Life!*

BAD HABITS THAT SHOW LACK OF SELF-ESTEEM

1. Saying "yes" to everything
2. Negative self-talk or self-criticism
3. Back down when opinions are challenged by others
4. Being indecisive with simple decisions
5. Fearing failure
6. Taking constructive criticism personally
7. Sweating the small stuff
8. Afraid to share your opinions in a conversation
9. Giving up too easily
10. Comparing yourself negatively to others
11. Slouching
12. Fidgeting
13. Claiming your successes are just luck
14. Buying things because others like them, not because you like them
15. Social withdrawal
16. Excessive preoccupation with personal problems
17. Letting fear stop you from trying new things

Affirm * Confirm * Claim Your Life!

Challenging Negative Thoughts

Automatic negative thoughts (ANTs) only have power to affect our mood and lives if we let them. Sometimes ANTs can make things seem like a bigger deal than they really are, and those negative thoughts can affect the way you perceive and react to the situation. It is important to know how to control ANTs so they do not control you. Next time you feel a negative emotion and feel yourself about to react, consider these questions:

What happened?

_____

_____

Why is this upsetting?

_____

_____

What is the negative thought? How does it make you feel?

_____

_____

How does what happened affect the next 5 minutes? 24 hours? 7 days?

_____

_____

How does what happened affect your quality of life?

_____

_____

How much power are you giving the negative thought?

_____

_____

Does that negative thought deserve the control it has over you?

_____

_____

Next time you have this negative thought, what will you remind yourself to stay in control?

_____

_____

*Affirm * Confirm * Claim Your Life!*

The Not-To-Do List

EVERYTHING ON MY PLATE	OTHER PEOPLE'S RESPONSIBILITIES
	STUFF THAT'S OUT OF MY CONTROL
	STUFF THAT DRAINS ME
	STUFF THAT DOESN'T NEED TO GET DONE

Affirm * Confirm * Claim Your Life!

Stress Diary
Finding Your Optimum Stress Levels:

Keeping a stress diary is an effective way of finding out what causes you stress, the level of stress you can handle and how you cope with stressors.

In your diary, write down your stress levels and how you feel throughout the day. In particular, notice "stressful" events. Record the following information:

- At least 5 times a day (on the hour - the same every day) write down:
    - The time
    - The amount of stress that you feel (on a scale of 1 to 10)
    - The emotions you are experiencing
    - How efficiently you think you are accomplishing things

- When you are feeling "stressed", write down:
    - Briefly describe the situation.
    - When and where did it occur?
    - What important factors made the event stressful?
    - Rate how stressful it was, on a scale of 1 to 10.
    - How did you handle the event?
    - Do you feel you handled the event well?
    - Did you deal with the cause or the symptom?
    - Overall, do you feel that you dealt with the stressor effectively?

*Affirm * Confirm * Claim Your Life!*

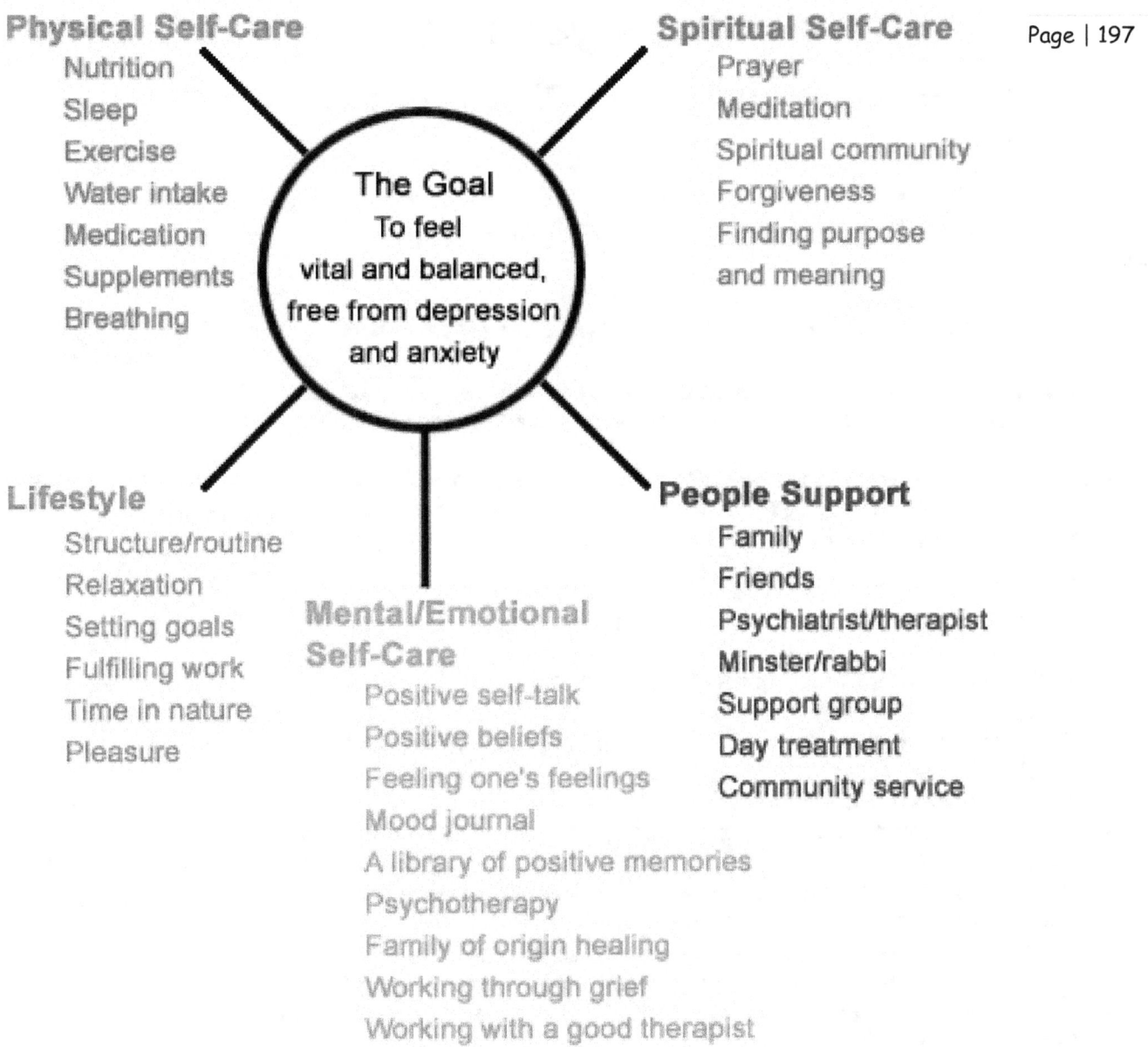

*Affirm * Confirm * Claim Your Life!*

Time Management
Organising Your Time & Plan Your Day

It's not possible to manage time because time doesn't actually exist. It is possible to organise your daily activities and make better use of the time that's available during the day.

PLAN YOUR TOMORROW AT THE END OF YOUR TODAY.

- If you are at work – plan your next day before you leave the workplace.
- If you are at home – plan your next day before going to sleep at night.

Take some time at the end of your day to finish up loose ends and focus on the priorities for the next day. Plan what needs to get done without overloading your schedule. If you have really important tasks that HAVE to be done - delegate time just for them.

It's not enough to be busy. The question is: "What are you busy about?"

Consider these questions when organising your tomorrow:

- What tasks need to be done to move forward in your project/goal?
- What is the best order for them to be done in?
- What tasks need to be done first?
- Which ones would you choose to be done tomorrow? The next day? Next week? Next month? And so on.
- When considering the tasks that need to be done tomorrow: Have you got enough time in the day to accomplish these tasks?
- Are there any tasks that you can delegate to another person?
- Do you need more information about a task before it can be completed?
- Are you more alert and at optimal potential in the morning or the afternoon? (Delegate tasks accordingly).
- What jobs or tasks are you forgetting?

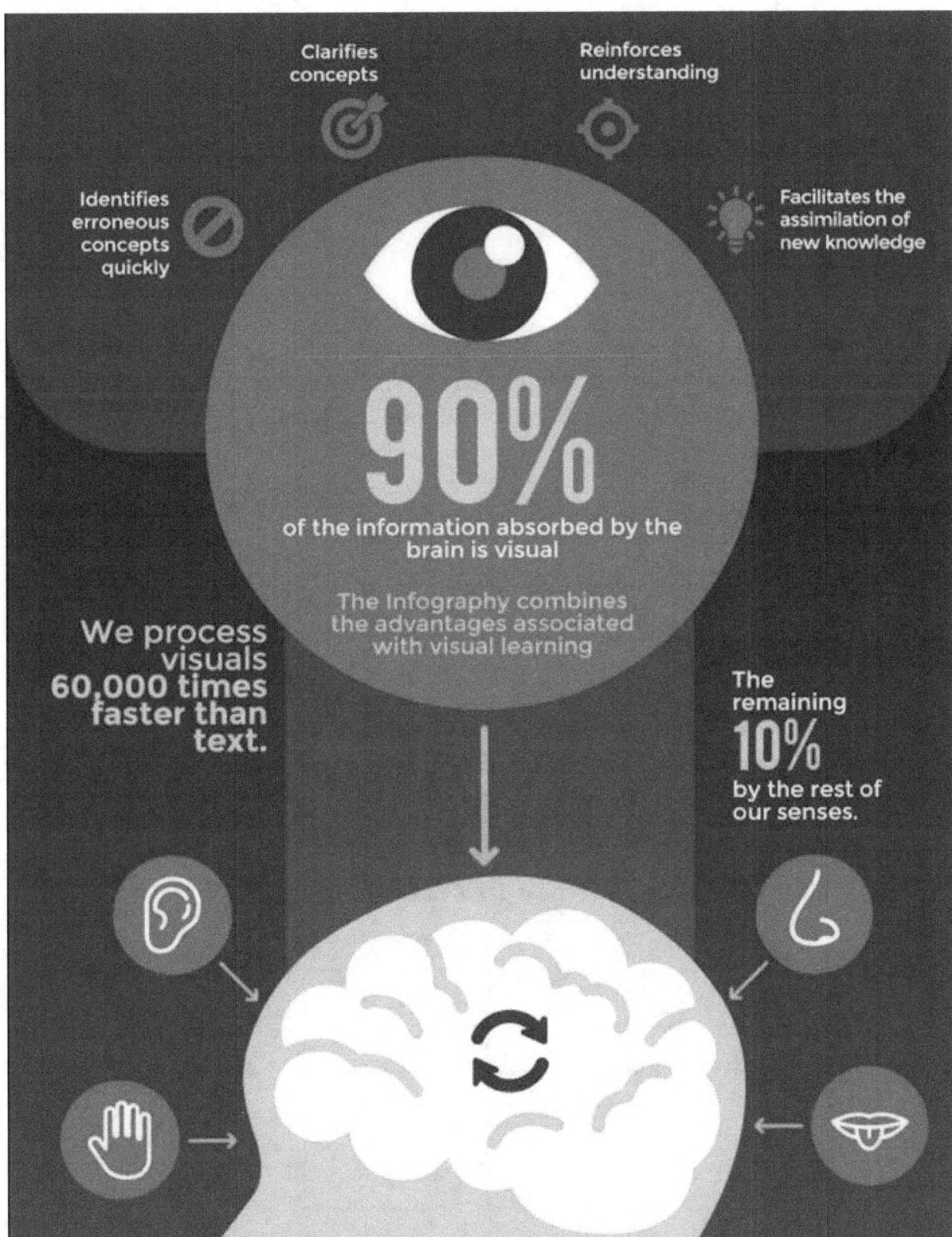

Affirm * Confirm * Claim Your Life!

Chapter Eleven

Achievement Motivation!

· · · · ·

Psychologists today define **motivation** as a need or desire that energizes and directs behavior. Our motivations arise from the interplay between nature (the bodily "**push**") and nurture (the "**pulls**" from our thought processes and culture).

Motivation a need or desire that energizes and directs behavior.

When there is both a need and an incentive, we feel strongly driven. You have a Need to Heal, a Need to become Healthy, a Need to become Powerful with a Strong incentive to Successfully Enjoy Your Abundant Life!!!

- **Achievement is reflected in stories about attaining challenging goals, setting new records, successful completion of difficult tasks, and doing something not done before.**

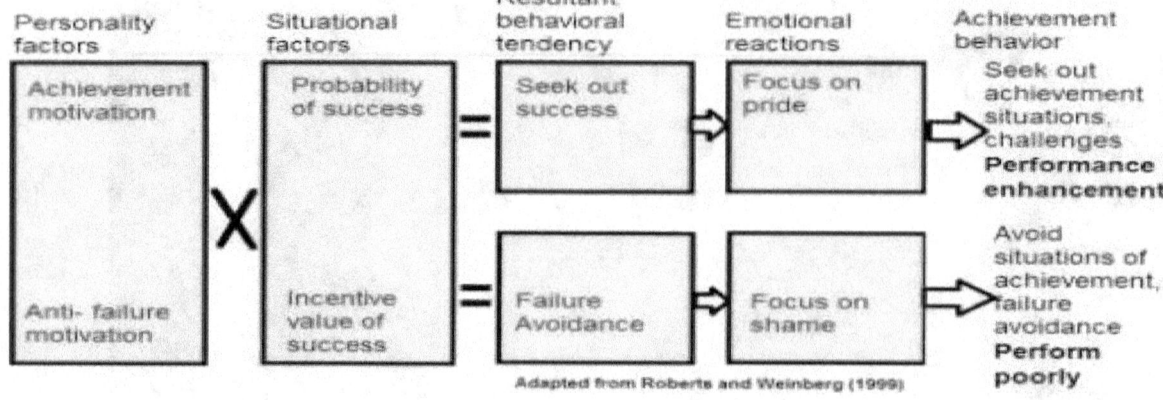

Affirm * Confirm * Claim Your Life!

What is achievement motivation?

The biological perspective on motivation—the idea that physiological needs drive us to satisfy those needs—provides only a partial explanation of what energizes and directs our behavior. Hunger and the need to belong have social as well as biological components.

Moreover, there are also motives that seem to have little obvious life orvsurvival value.

Billionaires may be motivated to make ever more money, movie stars to become ever more famous, politicians to achieve ever more power, daredevils to seek ever greater thrills. Such motives seem not to diminish when they are fed.

The more we achieve, the more we may need to achieve.

Think of someone you know who strives to succeed by excelling at any task where evaluation is possible. Now think of someone who is less driven.

Psychologist Henry Murray (1938) defined the first person's **achievement motivation** as a desire for significant accomplishment, for mastering skills or ideas, for control, and for rapidly attaining a high standard.

In this case, your Achievement Motivation is becoming One with YourSelf!

Your Achievement Motivation is to HEAL YOURSELF!!!!

Your Achievement Motivation is to make Manifest YOUR POWER!!!

Achievement Motivation a desire for significant accomplishment, for mastery of skills or ideas, for control, and for rapidly attaining a high standard.

As you might expect from their persistence and eagerness for realistic challenges, people with high achievement motivation do achieve more. One study followed the lives of 1528 California children whose intelligence test scores were in the top 1 percent. Forty years later, when researchers compared those who were most and least successful professionally, they found a motivational difference.

Those most successful were more ambitious, energetic, and persistent. As children, they had more active hobbies. As adults, they participated in more groups and favored being sports participants to being spectators (Goleman, 1980).

Gifted children are able learners. Accomplished adults are tenacious doers. Most of us are energetic doers when starting and finishing a project. It's easiest—have you noticed?—to "get stuck in the middle," which is when high achievers keep going (Bonezzi et al., 2011).

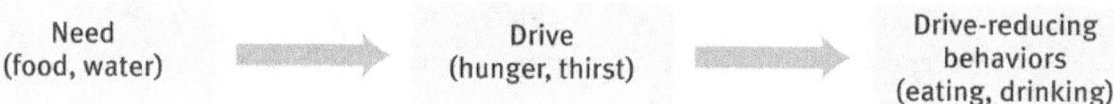

In their attempts to understand motivated behavior, psychologists have viewed it from four perspectives:

- **Instinct theory** (now replaced by the *evolutionary perspective*) focuses on genetically predisposed behaviors.

- **Drive-reduction theory** focuses on how we respond to our inner pushes.

- **Arousal theory** focuses on finding the right level of stimulation.

- Abraham Maslow's **hierarchy of needs** focuses on the priority of some needs over others.

ACHIEVEMENT MOTIVATION THEORY (contd..)

- Needs for achievement
- Needs for affiliation
- Needs for power

Power need (n Pow): this is the need to dominate, influence and control others. Power speaks about the ability to manipulate or control the activities of others to suit one's own purposes.

Affiliation need (n Aff): the need for affiliation is a social need, for companionship and support, for developing meaningful relationship with people.

Achievement need (n Ach): this is a need for challenge, for personal accomplishment and success in competitive situations.

Affirm * Confirm * Claim Your Life!

The physiological aim of drive reduction is **homeostasis**—the maintenance of a steady internal state. An example of homeostasis (literally "staying the same") is the body's temperature-regulation system, which works like a room's thermostat.

Both systems operate through feedback loops: Sensors feed room temperature to a control device. If the room's temperature cools, the control device switches on the furnace.

Likewise, if our body's temperature cools, our blood vessels constrict (to conserve warmth) and we feel driven to put on more clothes or seek a warmer environment.

Homeostasis a tendency to maintain a balanced or constant internal state; the regulation of any aspect of body chemistry, such as blood glucose, around a particular level.

Not only are we *pushed* by our need to reduce drives, we also are *pulled* by **incentives**—positive or negative environmental stimuli that lure or repel us. This is one way our individual learning histories influence our motives.

Depending on our learning, the aroma of good food, whether fresh roasted peanuts or toasted ants, can motivate our behavior. So can the sight of those we find attractive or threatening.

Incentive a positive or negative environmental stimulus that motivates behavior.

The Incentive in this Activity that we are using is coming from our Own self-generated Concepts, Visualizations and Love of self instead of an exogenous source.

Achievement Motivation

- Characteristics of those high in need for achievement
  - moderate risk takers
    - Avoid goals that are too easy or too hard
  - Complete difficult tasks
  - Earn better grades
  - Tend to excel in chosen occupations
  - Attribute success to ability; failure to insufficient effort
  - More likely to renew efforts when they perform poorly
- **Can you think of some disadvantages of a direct, objective test like this?**

Affirm * Confirm * Claim Your Life!

Setting Specific & Challenging Goals

In everyday life, our achievement goals sometimes involve approaching high levels of mastery or performance (such as mastering the material for this class and getting a high grade) and sometimes they involve avoiding failure (Elliot & McGregor, 2001).

In many situations, specific and/or challenging goals motivate and help facilitate our chance for achievement, (Johnson et al., 2006; Latham & Locke, 2007). When we set Specific, measurable objectives, such as "finish gathering the history paper information by Friday," they serve to direct our attention, promote our effort, motivate our persistence, and stimulate our creative strategies.

You are applying this science to YOURSELF!

The Specific Goal You are striving to Achieve is Your HEALING, Your LIFE, Your POWER and YOUR GREATNESS!

You will be applying the strategies to direct your Attention to Your Healing and POWER!

You will be employing these strategies to promote your Effort to DO the work that you need to create the environment IN you for your Healing and POWER!

You will be these strategies of your own words to provide the necessary Motivation of YOUR PERSISTENCE to make manifest Your HEALING and POWER!!!

When people state goals together with *subgoals* and *implementation intentions*—action plans that specify when, where, and how they will march toward achieving those goals—they become more focused in their work, and on-time completion becomes more likely (Burgess et al., 2004; Fishbach et al., 2006; Koestner et al., 2002).

Through a task's ups and downs, people best sustain their mood and motivation when they focus on immediate goals (such as daily study) rather than distant goals (such as a course grade). Better to have one's nose to the grindstone than one's eye on the ultimate prize (Houser-Marko & Sheldon, 2008).

Affirm * Confirm * Claim Your Life!

To motivate high productivity, effective leaders work with people to define explicit goals, sub-goals, and implementation plans, and then they provide feedback on progress.

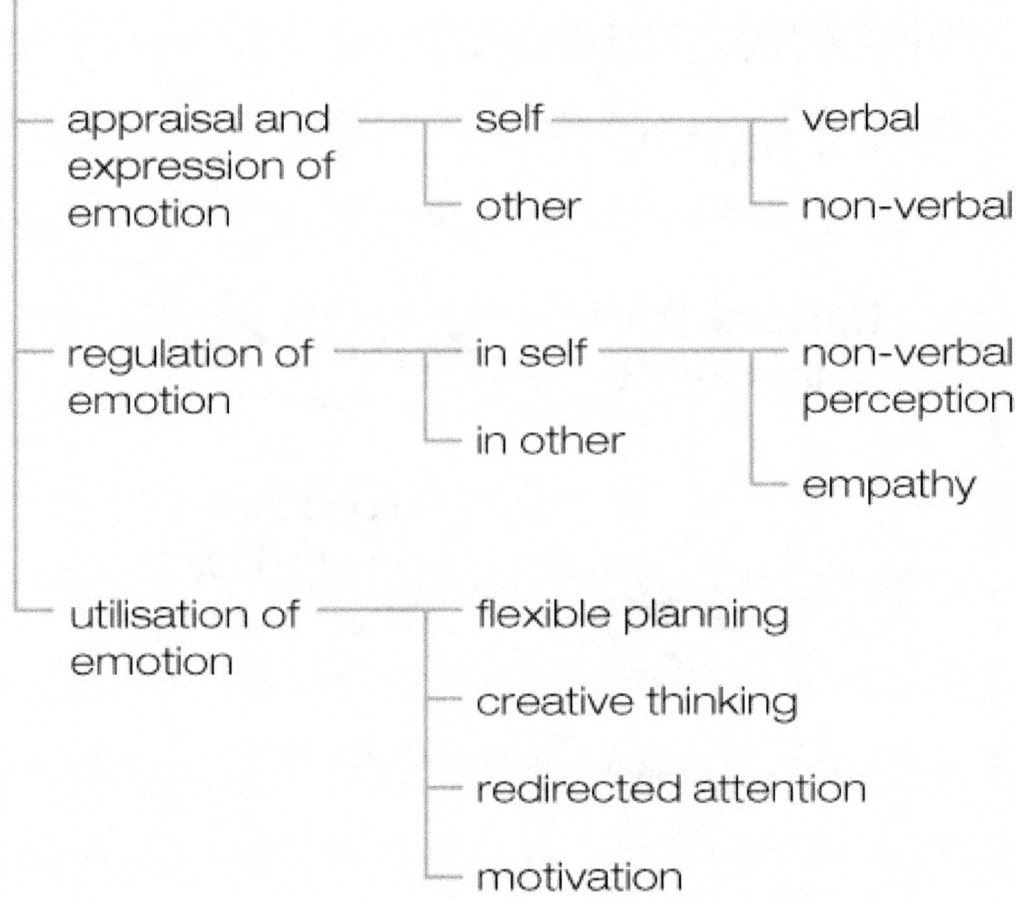

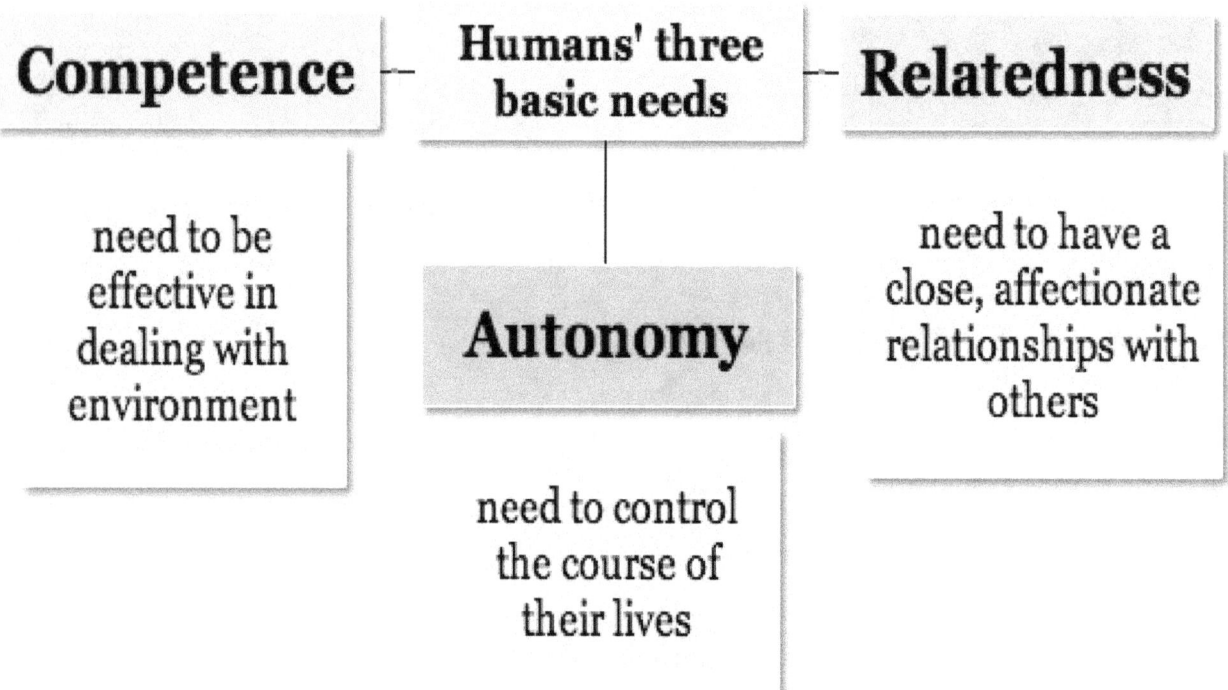

Characteristics of Expert Thought

Expertise is strategic

- Experts have more and better strategies, especially when problems are unexpected.

Expertise is flexible

- Experts are creative and curious, deliberately experimenting and enjoying the challenge when things do not go according to plan.

Outline

- **Mindsets**
- **Mindset 1: Deliberative-Implemental**
  - Deliberative mindset
  - Implemental mindset
  - Downstream consequences
- **Mindset 2: Promotion-Prevention**
  - Promotion Mindset
  - Prevention Mindset
  - Definitions of success and failure
  - Goal-striving strategies
  - Ideal and ought self-guides
  - Regulatory fit
- **Mindset 3: Growth-Fixed**
  - Fixed Mindset
  - Growth Mindset
  - Meaning of effort
  - Origins of fixed-growth motivation
  - Achievement goals
- **Mindset 4: Cognitive dissonance**
  - Dissonance-arousing situations
    - Choice
    - Insufficient justification
    - Effort justification
    - New information
  - Motivational processes
  - Self-perception theory

Brain-based Learning

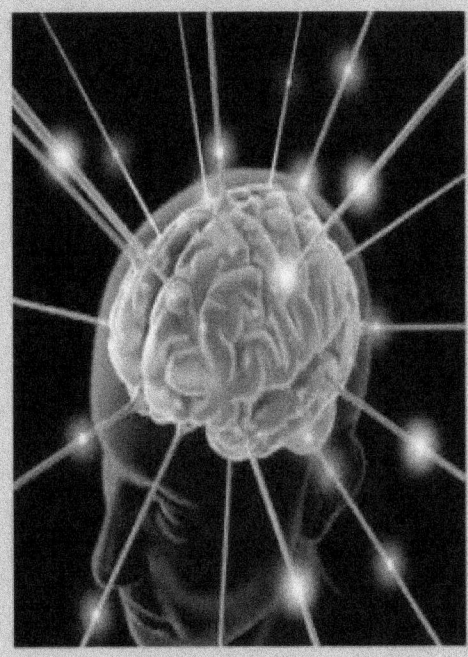

- is a theory based on the structure and function of the human brain. It constantly accessing information and interpreting its environment and continuously interacting with its surrounding to learn and how to function appropriately.

- Each brain is unique because it process information in ways that makes sense to the one brain may not make sense to another.

Affirm * Confirm * Claim Your Life!

Conclusion!

* * * * *

16 Ways to INCREASE Your God Energy!

We ARE WHAT WE THINK!

Thoughts are Vibrations.. Negative Thoughts Vibrate at a Low Frequency = Pre-Mature DEATH ... Positive Thoughts Vibrate at a HIGHER FREQUENCY = EVER-LASTING LIFE!

Vibrations can be influenced, slowed, interrupted, quickened.

The Vibrational Level of Thoughts Attracts it's Own Quality - Low Thoughts Attract Low Energy - HIGH Thoughts Attract HIGH Energy..!

When We RAISE our Thought Quality to that of GOD = INCREASING Our Vibrations to the HIGHEST LEVEL = ATTRACTING the Equivalent Levels Of God Energy OutSide of Self.

Then we Gain the Ability to SAY - BE & IT SHALL BE!

*EXERCISE!   +

*MEDITATION!   +

*AWARENESS of OutSide Vibrations!   +

*HYDRATION!   +

*BEING IN NATURE!   +

*EATING TO LIVE!   =

*Affirm * Confirm * Claim Your Life!*

RAISING OUR VIBRATION TO THAT OF GOD !

We are Created with the Abilities to LITERALLY SAY BE - AND IT SHALL BE !

Raise The Quality of Vibrations IN Self to that of GOD by Increasing your Thoughts Of GOD !!

Every THOUGHT produces an Equal Corresponding CHEMICAL HORMONE..

Thoughts of God Produces Chemical Hormones of God = Energy/Vibrations IN Self BECOME that Of GOD = BECOMING That THOUGHT of God !

SAY - BE & IT SHALL BECOME !!

THINK & BE THE GOD THAT YOU ARE !

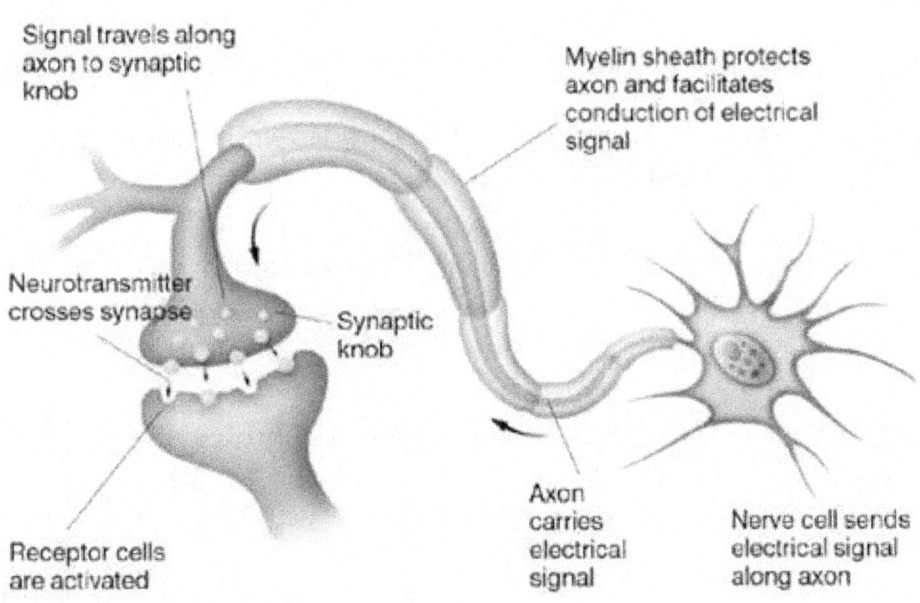

Affirm * Confirm * Claim Your Life!

PERFECTION IS ONLY AN IDEA/THOUGHT AWAY...!!

~~MATTHEW 5:48....BE you therefore PERFECT, even as your FATHER which is in Heaven is PERFECT...*King James Version!!*

~Therefore you are to BE PERFECT, as your Heavenly FATHER is PERFECT..... *New American Standard!!*

~That is WHY you MUST BE PERFECT as your FATHER in Heaven is PERFECT.... *GOD'S Word Translation!!*

HOW/WHY IS PERFECTION OBTAINABLE ??

~~Because we are Created IN the Image & Likeness of GOD !

What is PERFECT and/or Being PERFECT ?

~ PERFECT is expressed as an Adjective, Verb and Noun.

*As an Adjective, PERFECT means to have all the required or desirable Elements, Qualities or Characteristics - ANYONE of us can Fulfill this !

*As a Verb, PERFECT means to make something Completely FREE from faults or defects, or as close as possible = MUSLIM is the Act of Submission to ALLAH, which Frees us from Mental, Spiritual Enslavement

~PERFECTION is expressed as a Noun and means the condition, state or quality of being Free or Free as possible from flaws or defects = ISLAM - Surah 5:3.... 'This day have I PERFECTED for you your Religion...'

**Perfection also means the Action or Process of IMPROVING something until it is faultless, or as close as possible = SALAT/Prayer & Constant Training and Conditioning !

PERFECTIONIST is expressed as a Noun and Adjective.

Affirm * Confirm * Claim Your Life!

*As a Noun, PERFECTIONIST is One who REFUSES to accept any standard short of Perfect = A WIDE-AWAKE Man & Woman !

*As an Adjective, PERFECTIONIST means REFUSING to accept any Standard short of Perfect = we have the BEST STANDARD - The Sun, Moon & Star !

Each of Us are One-of-a-kind.... So Each of Us has a responsibility to BE Our Own PERFECT Self..!

We have a Perfect physical vehicle to Perfectly Manifest the God that We ARE !

We are Created with the Abilities to BE PERFECT and Manifest GOD !

We have a PERFECTED Way of LIFE in conjunction with an Order to BE Perfect..... Let Us be found Striving to BE the most PERFECT US WE CAN !

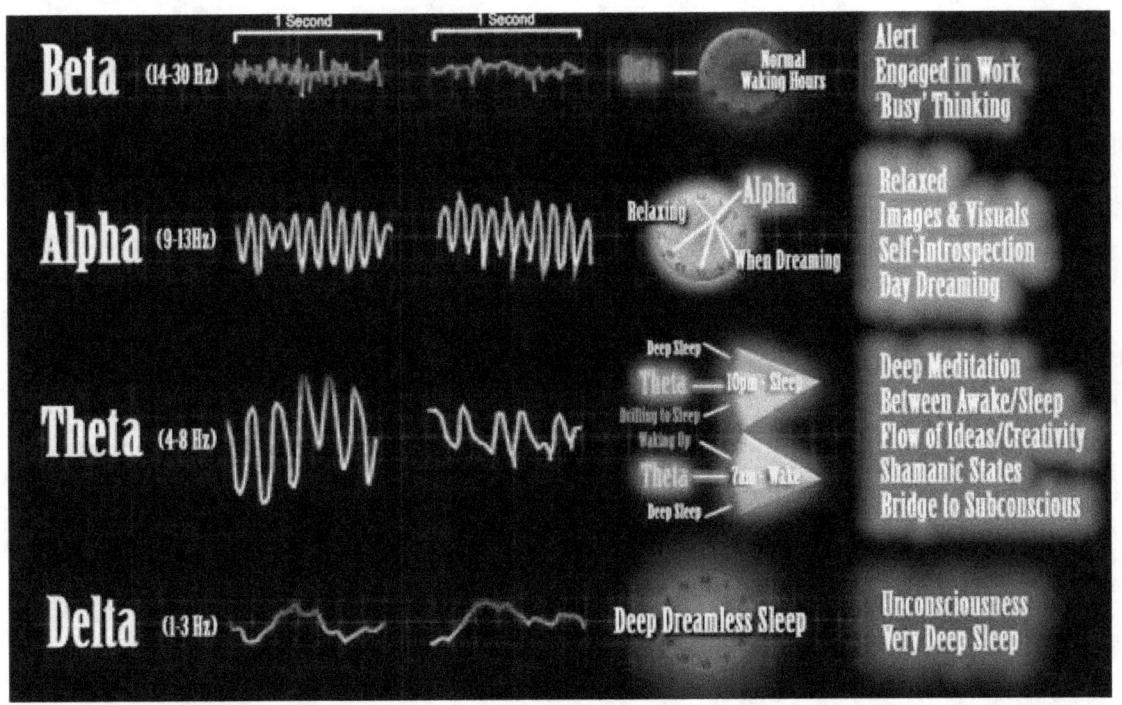

Affirm * Confirm * Claim Your Life!

Brain ENTRAINMENT - Building Your God With SOUNDS OF GOD!

We are Created with the Abilities to Move & Sustain Perpetual MOTION = EVER-LASTING LIFE !!

ALL LIFE is ENERGY..

ALL ENERGIES VIBRATE..

GOD HAS A SPECIFIC QUALITY OF VIBRATION..

We Can TUNE INTO that Level...

Vibrations & Sounds are the Same Sciences.. Sound being the Effects of Vibrations..

There are Sound Vibrations that can Harm = Decreases Atomic Rate of Rotation = Pre-Mature DEATH

Or

HEAL Us = INCREASES Atomic Rate of Rotation = PERPETUAL LIFE !

Our Bodies Constantly & Consistently Absorb & BECOME EVERY SOUND VIBRATION WE HEAR/FEEL..

That's Because All Matter VIBRATES = EVEN OUR CELLS. Our Cells are Constantly & Consistently RE-PRODUCING (Homeostasis).. This is an Act of Vibrations... So, OUTSIDE Sound Vibrations INFLUENCE Our Cell Reproduction = WE BECOME THAT SPECIFIC SOUND VIBRATION..

Our Cells Reproduce Approximately 300 Billion Cells EVERY 24 Hours..

So, depending on the Quality of Sound Vibrations = THE Quality Self will BE !

Affirm * Confirm * Claim Your Life!

The Higher/Chaotic the Sound Vibrations OUTSIDE = The MOST INTERFERENCE with CELLULAR Growth & Development by Reducing the amount of Human Growth Hormones (HGH).

The Higher/Chaotic the Sound Vibrations = the more dis-connect within the Cells.

The Higher/Chaotic the Sound Vibrations = the Activation of the AMYGDALA = Production of FEAR Hormones IN Self..   WHY CHILDREN DON'T LIKE LOUD NOISES..

The Lower/Peaceful the Sound Vibrations OUTSIDE of Self = HARMONY within the Cells = Normal Operating Procedures = HEALTHY SELF..

The Lower/Peaceful the Sound Vibrations = ACTIVATION of the PITUITARY GLAND = Enhanced Natural Production Human Growth Hormones = BUILDING GOD BODY !

It's as EASY AS LISTENING TO THE CORRECT TONES !!!

Turn the Radio, Tv, Phone, Computer OFF.. These project Vibrations that INTERFERE with Your Cellular RE-PRODUCTION = Un-Healthy Self !

Tune INTO the God Sound Vibrations = Lower/Peaceful Tones = Stimulate the PITUITARY Gland = Natural Production of Human Growth Hormones = BUILDING GOD BODY !

We are Created THIS WAY !

*Affirm * Confirm * Claim Your Life!*

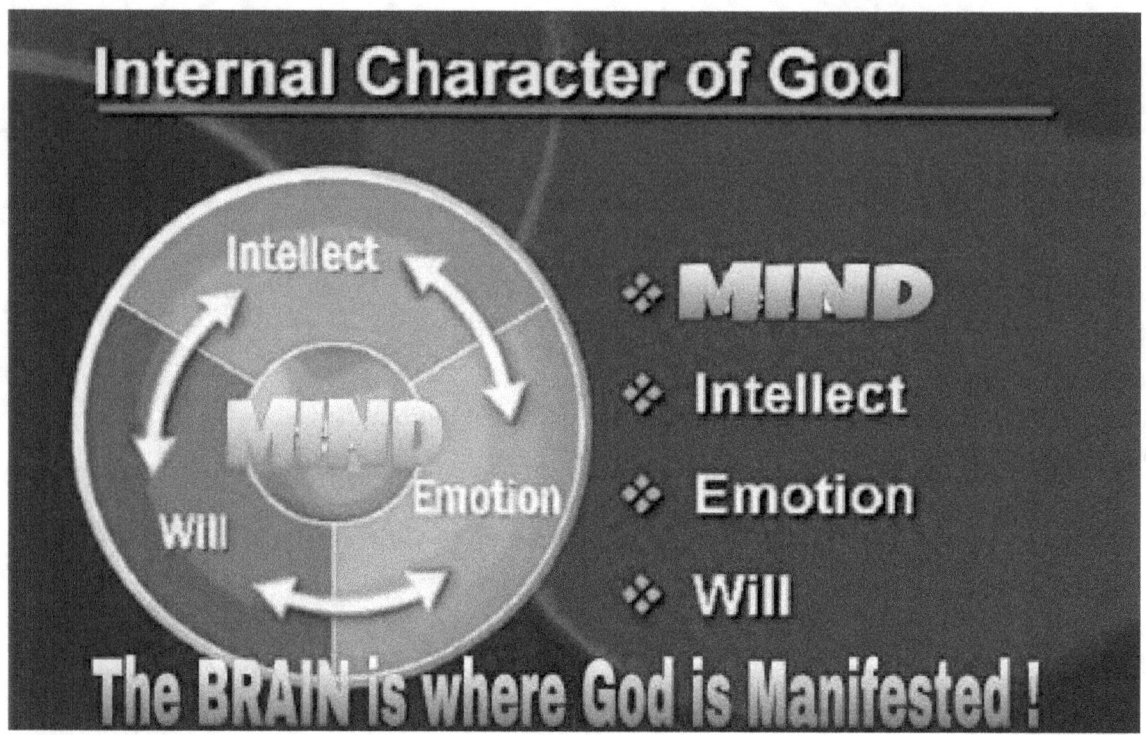

Building With Thought!

Every THOUGHT produces a Equal & Corresponding CHEMICAL HORMONE.

These Hormones are Neurotransmitters that Self Uses to Communicate With Self to Move Self.

Thoughts are Energy.

Low/Negative Thoughts/Energy produces A CATABOLIC Strength/Level of Energy.

This is LOW ENERGY that Vibrates at a SLOW SPEED that is Self-Destructive.

High/RIGHTEOUS Thoughts/Energy Manifest on an ANABOLIC Strength/Level.

Affirm * Confirm * Claim Your Life!

This is HIGH ENERGY THAT VIBRATES AT TERRIFIC SPEEDS that are Strong Enough to REMOVE the RUST from Our RUSTY LOCKS = MINDS !

Constant & Consistent Study, Prayer & Meditation is HOW We KEEP OurSelves IN-Tune with Righteous Thoughts = Producing RIGHTEOUS CHEMICAL Hormones = BECOMING RIGHTEOUSNESS !

We are Created with the Abilities to LITERALLY THINK into Existence that which we WANT & NEED.

Every THOUGHT (Un-Seen) produces a Equal CHEMICAL (Seen) Hormone that CREATES Self INTO THAT ANSWER/Solution to Our WANTS & NEEDS !

Constant & Consistent Submission to GOD = Prayer/Thought of God is = Producing God Hormones = GOD BODY !

Manifesting God !

We are Created with the Ability to THINK INTO EXISTENCE what we Need or Want.

We Believe IN God - BUT We Don't Believe IN BEING God !

We are Created in the Direct Express Image & Likeness of GOD.

We Simply Have to ACCEPT OUR OWN AND BE OURSELVES !

Our Thoughts CHEMICALLY begins to Create Self INTO the Thought.

The Production of God/Righteous Thoughts = Chemical Production of God/Righteous Hormones = BUILDING GOD BODY !

We have to Produce the Necessary Thoughts that Promotes the God THAT IS SELF !

These Thoughts create BELIEF IN THE GOD THAT IS SELF = BEING THE GOD THAT IS SELF !

*Affirm * Confirm * Claim Your Life!*

WE SIMPLY HAVE TO ACCEPT OUR OWN AND BE OURSELVES !

> "The greatest discovery of our generation is that human beings can alter their lives by altering their attitudes of mind. As you think, so shall you be."
> —William James

Knowledge of Self = KINGDOM OF GOD !

We are Ordered to SEEK 1ST THE KINGDOM OF GOD ..

That if We DO SO = ALL THINGS SHALL BE ADDED UNTO YOU!

Jesus was asked on this by the Pharisees of his Time as to the LOCATION of the KINGDOM OF GOD.

His ANSWER = IT IS IN YOU!!

Affirm * Confirm * Claim Your Life!

The Knowledge of Self = The KINGDOM OF GOD!

We are Created IN the Direct Express Image & Likeness of GOD!

We are Created with the Abilities to HAVE DOMINION OVER ALL ENERGIES/VIBRATIONS/LIFE!

These Capabilities COME WITH Seeking 1st of The KINGDOM OF GOD = Which is IN Self!

Becoming ONE with GOD is Becoming ONE with SELF!

THE KINGDOM OF GOD IS WITHIN YOU!

It is IN Self that We FIND GOD = THE MIND!

The MIND is where The ABILITY to THINK of GOD & REALIZE GOD Lays.

The MIND is the ACTIVE Control of the BRAIN.

We are Created with a IN-VOLUNTARY Muscle System and an AUTONOMIC Nervous System that KEEPS SELF ALIVE ON IT'S OWN!

When We STUDY Self - We FIND that We have a Limited Control of Self = VOLUNTARY MUSCLE System.

This ALLOWS Us to Move Self BEYOND the Basic FUNCTIONS & MANIFEST GOD = Dominion Over ALL Energies/Vibrations/Life!

THE KINGDOM OF GOD IS WITHIN YOU!

SEEK YOU 1ST THE KINGDOM OF GOD (SELF) & ALL THESE THINGS SHALL BE ADDED UNTO YOU!

*Affirm * Confirm * Claim Your Life!*

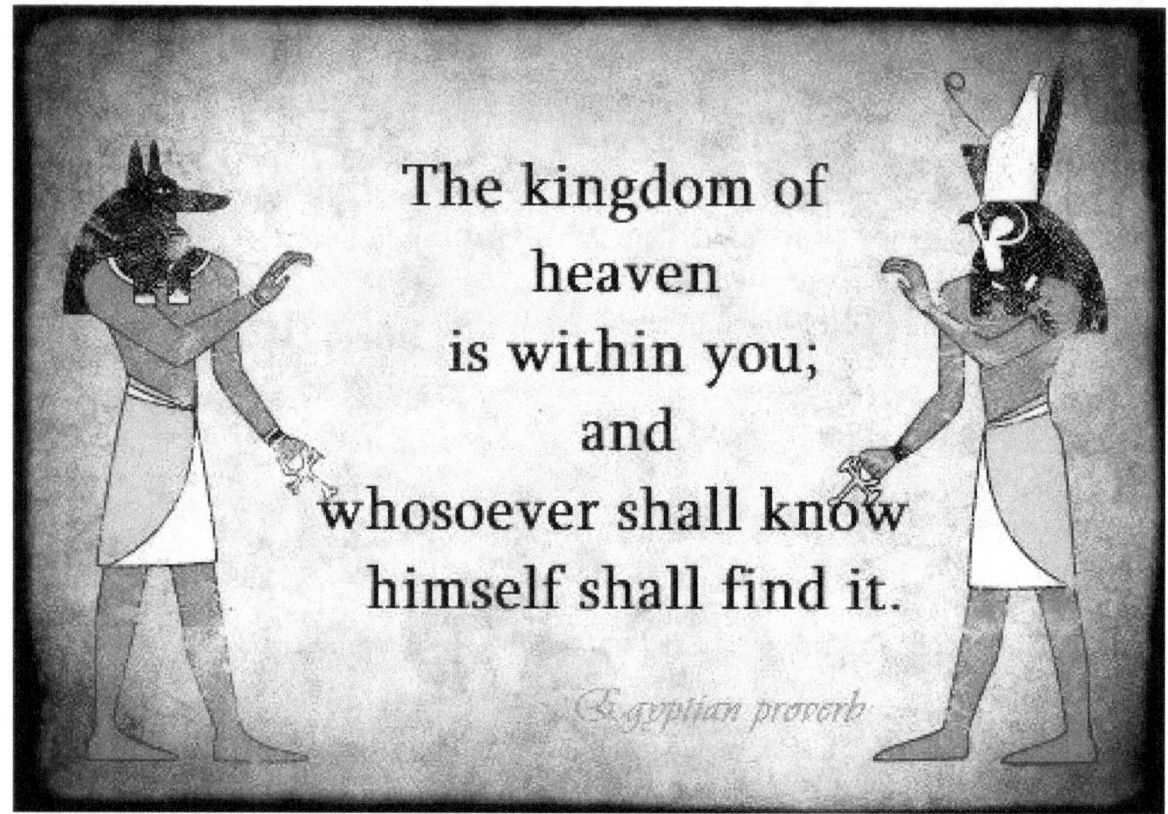

The Power of Prayer & Fasting!

We were Taught by Jesus that the KINGDOM OF GOD IS WITHIN SELF ..

SO, WHERE IS THAT STRAIGHT PATH TO BECOME ONE WITH GOD LOCATED??

ALL WE HAVE TO DO IS LOOK IN SELF ALSO!!

At the Top of the Spinal Column is the BRAIN - the Power Center - WHERE we BEcome ONE with GOD..

At the Bottom is the Digestive & Reproductive Organs - the Power Center of Appetite & Desires - Where we Lose Touch with GOD.

*Affirm * Confirm * Claim Your Life!*

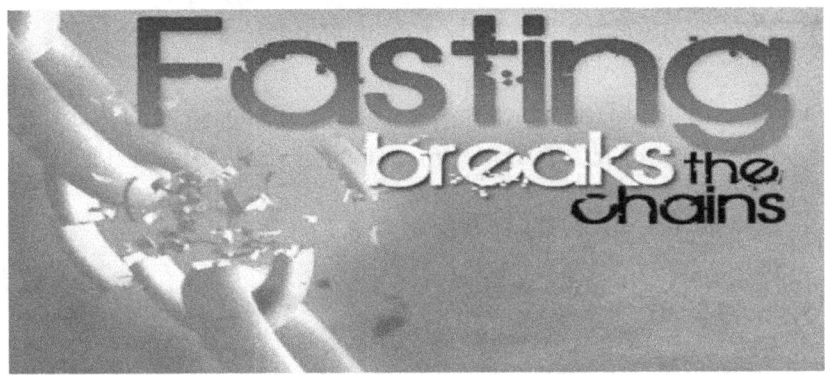

We are Created with the Abilities to Produce a Thought & LITERALLY Manifest that Thought by BECOMING THAT THOUGHT!

Thoughts are Un-Seen Energy/Vibrations that Produces the Equivalent in a SEEN CHEMICAL HORMONE.

Thoughts are of Varying Degrees & Qualities.

GOD, PRAYER, LOVE, CHARITY and HELPING Others are Examples of Higher Quality Thoughts.

**These Levels of Thoughts Produce Chemical Hormones that ACTIVATE THE BRAIN - The POWER Center of Self = Obtaining MAXIMUM Power of Self ..

**This is HOW we Manifest Righteousness, Unity and Love ..

**With Our Power Located in the Brain = The Force & Power to Manifest God.

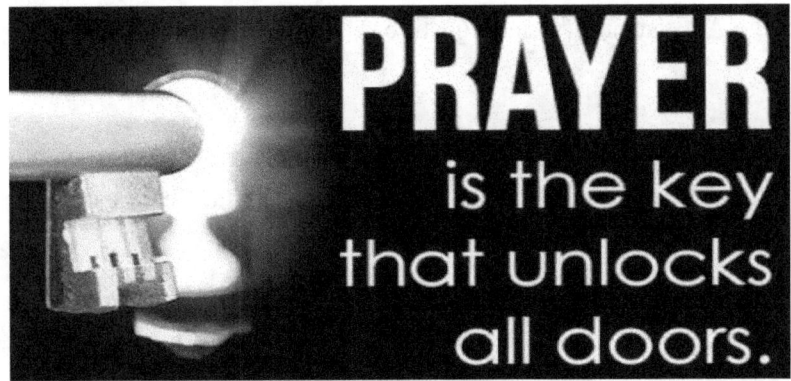

HUNGER, LUST, DESIRES and ANGER are Examples of Low Quality Thoughts.

**These Levels of Thought Produces Chemical Hormones that Activate the Digestive or Reproductive Organs = De-Activates the Power in the Brain/Power Center = MINIMAL Power of Self.

**This is HOW Un-Righteousness, Dis-Unity, Hatred is Made.

**With the Power Located in the Digestive or Reproductive Organs = We move to SATISFY the Hunger/Lust/Desires... The Brain is at Minimum Power as these Organs Move Self to Fulfill that Low Thought.

PRAYER & FASTING!

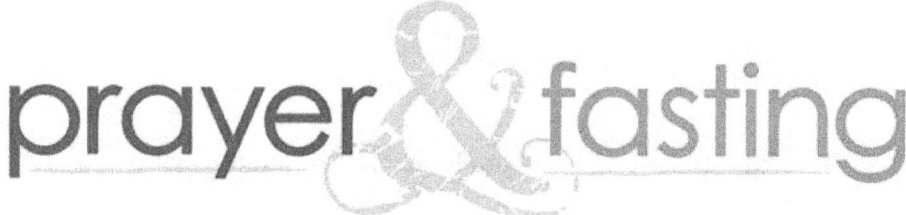

Prayer & Fasting are the Catalyst for Mastery of Keeping Power in the Brain by Allowing Self-Control OVER APPETITES & DESIRES ..

PRAYER is at the Highest Quality of Thoughts.

+

FASTING is the Abstaining from the Activation of The Digestive & Reproductive Organs.

=

Power STAYS IN THE BRAIN = Maximum Control of Self = ABILITY to Manifest God!

Affirm * Confirm * Claim Your Life!

> **Proverbs 12:18 "There is one whose rash words are like sword thrusts, but the tongue of the wise brings healing."**

Speaking Grammatically Correct In Perfect Tense!

WHY We MUST Speak and Use Grammatic Pronunciation of Words and Syllables in Past, Future, Present and PERFECT TENSE = REMOVING THE RUST OFF OUR PEOPLE'S MIND = FREEDOM = BEING GOD!

We Know that we have been made Other-than-Self..

We know that the Knowledge of Self has been stripped & that any remnants have been RUSTED Over by Constant Re-defining of Us by Others..

All LIFE is ENERGY..

ALL ENERGIES VIBRATE!

VIBRATION IS THE MOST EFFECTIVE WAY TO REMOVE RUST!

We are Ordered to Speak in the Past, Future, Present and Perfect Tense..

We are ASKED WHAT IS MEANT by Answering the Lessons in the Past, Present & Future being PERFECT.

Achieving the PERFECTED VIBRATIONAL Level to Remove the Rust off the Mind IS THE ANSWER!

We all VIBRATE. We Project Our Vibrations WITH our WORDS!

We can ONLY Project the Level & Quality of Vibrations that We ARE..

Affirm * Confirm * Claim Your Life!

So, having an Answer in the Past, Present & Future Tense = Projecting Words/Vibrations/Energy in the Past, Present & Future PERFECT TENSE = Destroying devil & BUILDING GOD !

But WE MUST LOVE!

GOD IS LOVE..

GOD & LOVE ARE THE HIGHEST QUALITY OF VIBRATIONS/ENERGY.!

Having a Knowledge of GOD Creates LOVE OF & IN Self.. We SEE Our People AS SELF = LOVE OF PEOPLE/SELF..

When have the Necessary Presence of LOVE for Our People = Project Words of God/Love = REMOVING THE RUST OFF THE MIND!

THE TRUE LOVE OF SELF = THE TRUE LOVE OF OUR PEOPLE !

Our People have been Un-Loved, Abused, Mis-Treated.. And Want ONLY TO BE LOVED!!

If we Speak in the Past, Present and Future PERFECT TENSE = Speaking with LOVE = Projecting the Highest Quality of Vibrations = ABILITY to Remove the RUST off Our Minds = BUILDING GOD!

the **power** of words can move you to tears, evoke absolute joy or lead you in action. there are words of encouragement, of sympathy, of love & admiration. the right words can give you **strength**, define your *faith*, give flight to things that live in your **imagination**. Words will inspire you, cut you, bring you back to life. They will comfort you in your time of need. words will **nourish your soul.**

Affirm * Confirm * Claim Your Life!

A strong positive mental attitude will create more miracles than any wonder drug.

Man, Know ThySelf..... GOD, HEAL THYSELF!!!!

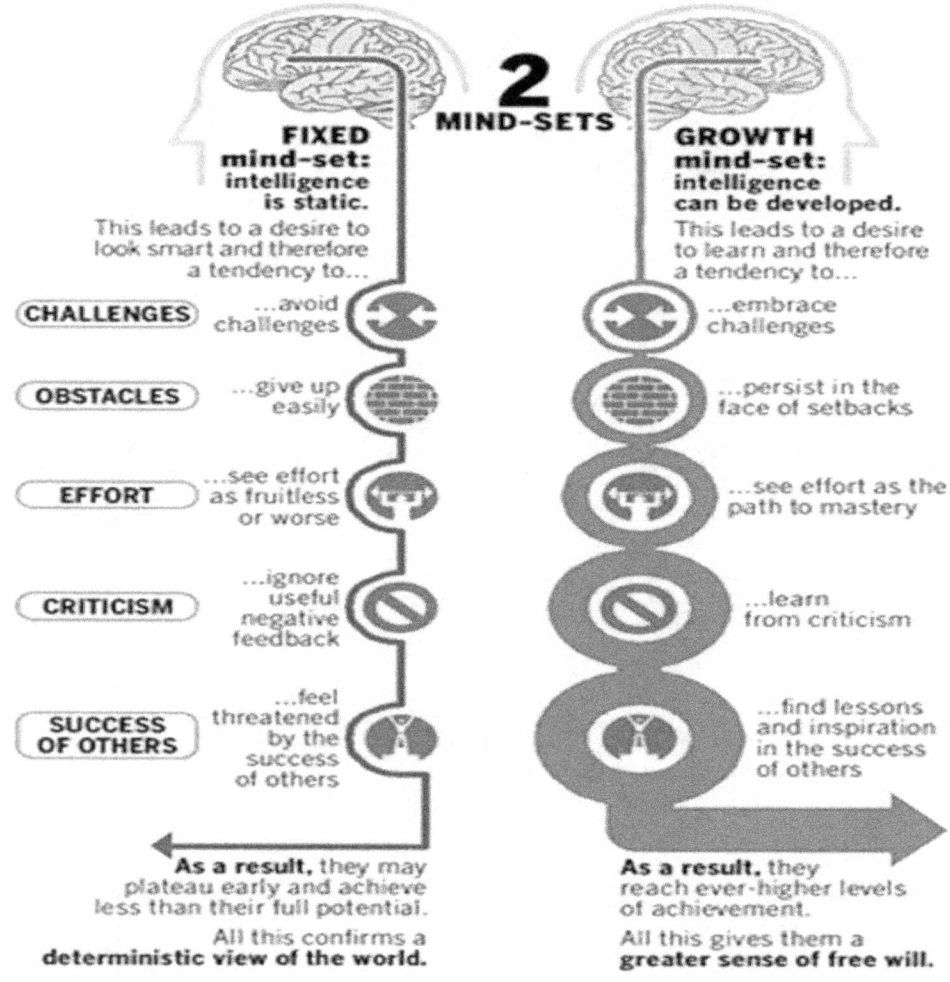

*Affirm * Confirm * Claim Your Life!*

Goals for Your Mind Body & Soul

GOALS FOR MY MIND, BODY & SOUL

- GOALS FOR MY MIND
- GOALS FOR MY BODY
- GOALS FOR MY SOUL

*Affirm * Confirm * Claim Your Life!*

Goals for Your Mind Body & Soul

GOALS FOR MY MIND, BODY & SOUL

- GOALS FOR MY MIND
- GOALS FOR MY BODY
- GOALS FOR MY SOUL

*Affirm * Confirm * Claim Your Life!*

DAILY DEVOTIONAL WORKSHEET
DATE:

SCRIPTURE VERSE THAT SPOKE TO ME

THINK QUALITY, NOT QUANTITY.

☐ BOOM. MEMORIZED IT.

WORD STUDY FROM MY SCRIPTURE VERSE

PRAYING THE SCRIPTURE

PERSONALIZE IT & TURN IT INTO A PRAYER.

DISTRACTION PARKING LOT

JOT IT DOWN & YOU'LL GET TO IT LATER.

MEDITATION

JOURNAL A THOUGHT OR TWO.

Supreme Health & Fitness!   Knowledge Of Self Series Vol 2!

*Affirm * Confirm * Claim Your Life!*

DAILY DEVOTIONAL WORKSHEET
DATE:

SCRIPTURE VERSE THAT SPOKE TO ME

THINK QUALITY, NOT QUANTITY.

☐ **BOOM. MEMORIZED IT.**

WORD STUDY FROM MY SCRIPTURE VERSE

PRAYING THE SCRIPTURE

PERSONALIZE IT & TURN IT INTO A PRAYER.

DISTRACTION PARKING LOT

JOT IT DOWN & YOU'LL GET TO IT LATER.

MEDITATION

JOURNAL A THOUGHT OR TWO.

Supreme Health & Fitness! Knowledge Of Self Series Vol 2!

*Affirm * Confirm * Claim Your Life!*

DAILY DEVOTIONAL WORKSHEET
DATE:

SCRIPTURE VERSE THAT SPOKE TO ME

THINK QUALITY, NOT QUANTITY.

☐ **BOOM. MEMORIZED IT.**

WORD STUDY FROM MY SCRIPTURE VERSE

PRAYING THE SCRIPTURE

PERSONALIZE IT & TURN IT INTO A PRAYER.

DISTRACTION PARKING LOT

JOT IT DOWN & YOU'LL GET TO IT LATER.

MEDITATION

JOURNAL A THOUGHT OR TWO.

Supreme Health & Fitness!   Knowledge Of Self Series Vol 2!

*Affirm * Confirm * Claim Your Life!*

DAILY DEVOTIONAL WORKSHEET
DATE:

SCRIPTURE VERSE THAT SPOKE TO ME

THINK QUALITY, NOT QUANTITY.

☐ **BOOM. MEMORIZED IT.**

WORD STUDY FROM MY SCRIPTURE VERSE

PRAYING THE SCRIPTURE

PERSONALIZE IT & TURN IT INTO A PRAYER.

DISTRACTION PARKING LOT

JOT IT DOWN & YOU'LL GET TO IT LATER.

MEDITATION

JOURNAL A THOUGHT OR TWO.

Supreme Health & Fitness!   Knowledge Of Self Series Vol 2!

Repeat after me....

I am Amazing and Astonishing.
I am Brilliant and Beautiful.
I am Clever, Courageous and Caring.
I am fabulous, Funny and Giving.
I am Happy, Loving and Loveable.
I am Outstanding and Sexy.
I am Terrific, Tantalising and
Totally Wonderful.
I am Unique and Special and
most importantly
I am ME.
ok great now say it again...
   by build your confidence.

Repetition

- Repetition is necessary to reinforce the neural pathways
- It strengthens long-term memory
- It facilitates transfer from short-term to long-term memory

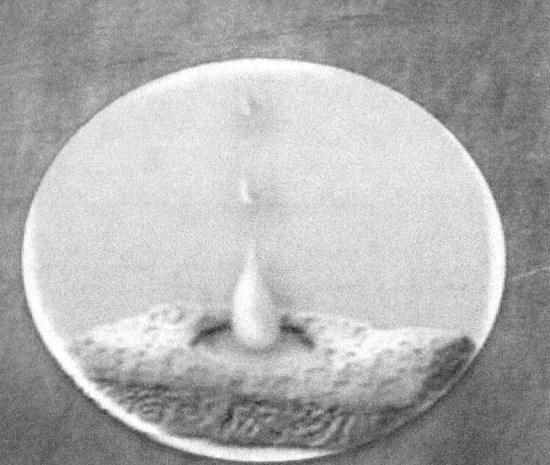

Difference between Intelligence and Learning Styles

- Intelligences are areas which we are more proficient at
- Learning styles are how we process information
- Intelligences affect learning styles
- Skills can be learned to compensate for weaknesses
- Intelligences and weaknesses change over time with experiences.

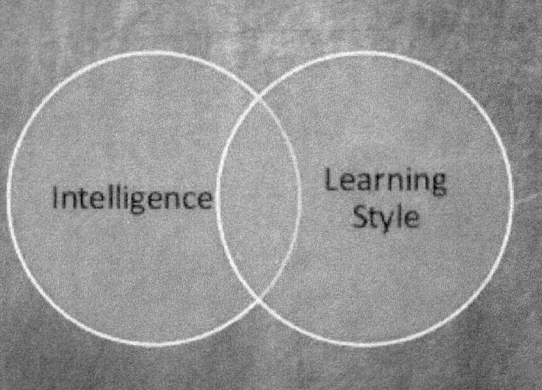

*Affirm * Confirm * Claim Your Life!*

My Strengths and Qualities

Things I am good at:
1. _____
2. _____
3. _____

Compliments I have received:
1. _____
2. _____
3. _____

What I like about my appearance:
1. _____
2. _____
3. _____

Challenges I have overcome:
1. _____
2. _____
3. _____

I've helped others by:
1. _____
2. _____
3. _____

Things that make me unique:
1. _____
2. _____
3. _____

What I value the most:
1. _____
2. _____
3. _____

Times I've made others happy:
1. _____
2. _____
3. _____

Supreme Health & Fitness!

Affirm * Confirm * Claim Your Life!

Positivity Pledge

I shall no longer allow negative
thoughts or feelings
to drain me of my energy.
Instead I shall focus on all the
good that is in my life.
I will think it, feel it and speak it.
By doing so I will send out
vibes of positive energy into
the world and I shall be grateful
for all the wonderful things it
will attract into my life.

*Affirm * Confirm * Claim Your Life!*

Reflection

Date: _____

This week I did / did not make my goal. Why?

_____
_____
_____
_____
_____
_____

Overall, I would rate my effort towards my goal: ☺   😐   ☹

Next Steps:

_____
_____
_____

"A goal without a plan is just a wish."

Supreme Health & Fitness!   Knowledge Of Self Series Vol 2!

*Affirm * Confirm * Claim Your Life!*

Reflection

Date: _____

This week I did / did not make my goal. Why?

_____
_____
_____
_____
_____

Overall, I would rate my effort towards my goal: ☺   😐   ☹

Next Steps:

_____
_____
_____

"A goal without a plan is just a wish."

Supreme Health & Fitness!   Knowledge Of Self Series Vol 2!

*Affirm * Confirm * Claim Your Life!*

Reflection

Date: _____

This week I did / did not make my goal. Why?

_____
_____
_____
_____
_____
_____

Overall, I would rate my effort towards my goal: 😊   😐   ☹

Next Steps:

_____
_____
_____

"A goal without a plan is just a wish."

*Affirm * Confirm * Claim Your Life!*

Reflection

Date: _____

This week I did / did not make my goal. Why?

_____
_____
_____
_____
_____

Overall, I would rate my effort towards my goal: ☺   😐   ☹

Next Steps:

_____
_____
_____

"A goal without a plan is just a wish."

Supreme Health & Fitness!   Knowledge Of Self Series Vol 2!

Affirm * Confirm * Claim Your Life!

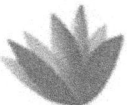 # Aspiration Journal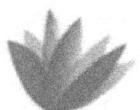

An aspiration journal is where you write AS IF everything you want to happen in your day, week, month, year, or life has already happened. If you want a new job, don't write "I wish I had a new job." Instead, write "I love my job as Marketing Manager, and I feel so good to be sitting at my big desk in my corner office. I'm respected and liked by all my colleagues." This way you can tap into the positive feelings related to what you want and start attracting those good things to you.

ALL THE GOOD THINGS THAT HAPPENED TODAY

THE ONE THING THAT MAKES ME HAPPIEST

HOW TODAY MAKES ME FEEL

*Affirm * Confirm * Claim Your Life!*

ALL THE GOOD THINGS THAT HAPPENED TODAY

THE ONE THING THAT MAKES ME HAPPIEST

HOW TODAY MAKES ME FEEL

*Affirm * Confirm * Claim Your Life!*

ALL THE GOOD THINGS THAT HAPPENED TODAY

THE ONE THING THAT MAKES ME HAPPIEST

HOW TODAY MAKES ME FEEL

*Affirm * Confirm * Claim Your Life!*

ALL THE GOOD THINGS THAT HAPPENED TODAY

THE ONE THING THAT MAKES ME HAPPIEST

HOW TODAY MAKES ME FEEL

Supreme Health & Fitness! Knowledge Of Self Series Vol 2!

Affirm * Confirm * Claim Your Life!

daily Self love Worksheets

DATE:

I **LOVE** MYSELF TODAY BECAUSE _

TODAY I FORGIVE MYSELF THAT _

I AM _____ BECAUSE _

SOMETHING GOOD I DID FOR MYSELF TODAY:

NOTES

DATE:

I **LOVE** MYSELF TODAY BECAUSE _

TODAY I FORGIVE MYSELF THAT _

I AM _____ BECAUSE _

SOMETHING GOOD I DID FOR MYSELF TODAY:

NOTES

*Affirm * Confirm * Claim Your Life!*

daily Self love Worksheets

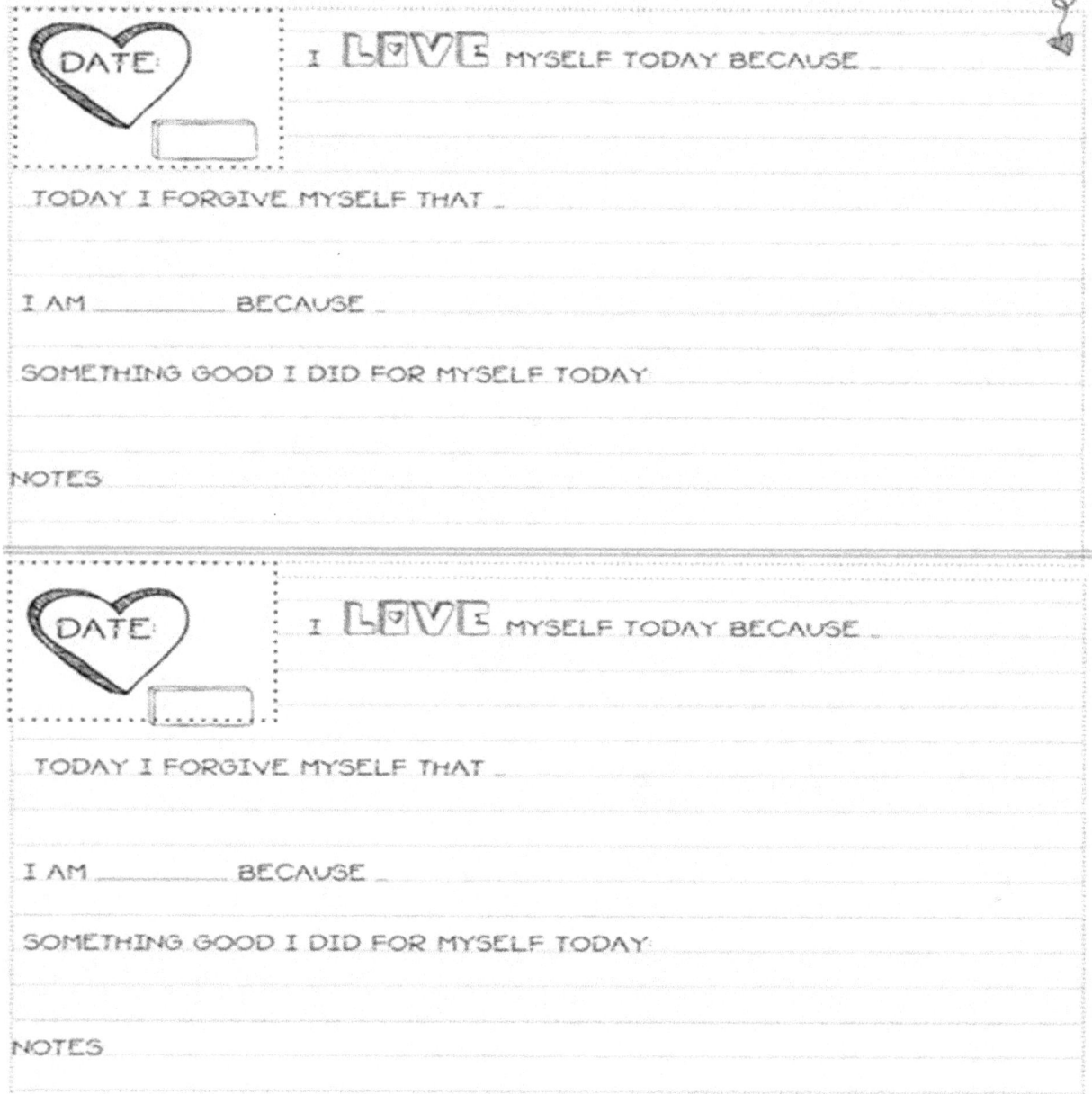

DATE:

I LOVE MYSELF TODAY BECAUSE _

TODAY I FORGIVE MYSELF THAT _

I AM _____ BECAUSE _

SOMETHING GOOD I DID FOR MYSELF TODAY:

NOTES

DATE:

I LOVE MYSELF TODAY BECAUSE _

TODAY I FORGIVE MYSELF THAT _

I AM _____ BECAUSE _

SOMETHING GOOD I DID FOR MYSELF TODAY:

NOTES

*Affirm * Confirm * Claim Your Life!*

daily Self love Worksheets

DATE:

I LOVE MYSELF TODAY BECAUSE

TODAY I FORGIVE MYSELF THAT

I AM _____ BECAUSE

SOMETHING GOOD I DID FOR MYSELF TODAY

NOTES

DATE:

I LOVE MYSELF TODAY BECAUSE

TODAY I FORGIVE MYSELF THAT

I AM _____ BECAUSE

SOMETHING GOOD I DID FOR MYSELF TODAY

NOTES

*Affirm * Confirm * Claim Your Life!*

daily Self love Worksheets

DATE:

I LOVE MYSELF TODAY BECAUSE ...

TODAY I FORGIVE MYSELF THAT ...

I AM _____ BECAUSE ...

SOMETHING GOOD I DID FOR MYSELF TODAY

NOTES

DATE:

I LOVE MYSELF TODAY BECAUSE ...

TODAY I FORGIVE MYSELF THAT ...

I AM _____ BECAUSE ...

SOMETHING GOOD I DID FOR MYSELF TODAY

NOTES

*Affirm * Confirm * Claim Your Life!*

Self-Esteem Journal

MON.	Something I did well today...	
	Today I had fun when...	
	I felt proud when...	
TUE.	Today I accomplished...	
	I had a positive experience with...	
	Something I did for someone...	
WED.	I felt good about myself when...	
	I was proud of someone else...	
	Today was interesting because...	
THUR.	I felt proud when...	
	A positive thing I witnessed...	
	Today I accomplished...	
FRI.	Something I did well today...	
	I had a positive experience with (a person, place, or thing)...	
	I was proud of someone when...	
SAT.	Today I had fun when...	
	Something I did for someone...	
	I felt good about myself when...	
SUN.	A positive thing I witnessed...	
	Today was interesting because...	
	I felt proud when...	

Supreme Health & Fitness!   Knowledge Of Self Series Vol 2!

*Affirm * Confirm * Claim Your Life!*

Self-Esteem Journal

MON.	Something I did well today...	
	Today I had fun when...	
	I felt proud when...	
TUE.	Today I accomplished...	
	I had a positive experience with...	
	Something I did for someone...	
WED.	I felt good about myself when...	
	I was proud of someone else...	
	Today was interesting because...	
THUR.	I felt proud when...	
	A positive thing I witnessed...	
	Today I accomplished...	
FRI.	Something I did well today...	
	I had a positive experience with (a person, place, or thing)...	
	I was proud of someone when...	
SAT.	Today I had fun when...	
	Something I did for someone...	
	I felt good about myself when...	
SUN.	A positive thing I witnessed...	
	Today was interesting because...	
	I felt proud when...	

Supreme Health & Fitness!   *Knowledge Of Self Series Vol 2!*

Affirm * Confirm * Claim Your Life!

Self-Esteem Journal

MON.	Something I did well today...	
	Today I had fun when...	
	I felt proud when...	
TUE.	Today I accomplished...	
	I had a positive experience with...	
	Something I did for someone...	
WED.	I felt good about myself when...	
	I was proud of someone else...	
	Today was interesting because...	
THUR.	I felt proud when...	
	A positive thing I witnessed...	
	Today I accomplished...	
FRI.	Something I did well today...	
	I had a positive experience with (a person, place, or thing)...	
	I was proud of someone when...	
SAT.	Today I had fun when...	
	Something I did for someone...	
	I felt good about myself when...	
SUN.	A positive thing I witnessed...	
	Today was interesting because...	
	I felt proud when...	

Supreme Health & Fitness!   Knowledge Of Self Series Vol 2!

*Affirm * Confirm * Claim Your Life!*

Self-Esteem Journal

MON.	Something I did well today...	
	Today I had fun when...	
	I felt proud when...	
TUE.	Today I accomplished...	
	I had a positive experience with...	
	Something I did for someone...	
WED.	I felt good about myself when...	
	I was proud of someone else...	
	Today was interesting because...	
THUR.	I felt proud when...	
	A positive thing I witnessed...	
	Today I accomplished...	
FRI.	Something I did well today...	
	I had a positive experience with (a person, place, or thing)...	
	I was proud of someone when...	
SAT.	Today I had fun when...	
	Something I did for someone...	
	I felt good about myself when...	
SUN.	A positive thing I witnessed...	
	Today was interesting because...	
	I felt proud when...	

Supreme Health & Fitness!   Knowledge Of Self Series Vol 2!

Affirm * Confirm * Claim Your Life!

Daily Food Diary for : _____

Food Group	Food Name and Amount
Breakfast	
Grains/Starches	
Vegetables	
Fruits	
Dairy	
Protein	
Fats/Sweets	
Beverages	
Comments	
Snack	
Lunch	
Grains/Starches	
Vegetables	
Fruits	
Dairy	
Protein	
Fats/Sweets	
Beverages	
Comments	
Snack	
Dinner	
Grains/Starches	
Vegetables	
Fruits	
Dairy	
Protein	
Fats/Sweets	
Beverages	
Comments	

*Affirm * Confirm * Claim Your Life!*

Daily Food Diary for _____

Food Group	Food Name and Amount
Breakfast	
Grains/Starches	
Vegetables	
Fruits	
Dairy	
Protein	
Fats/Sweets	
Beverages	
Comments	
Snack	
Lunch	
Grains/Starches	
Vegetables	
Fruits	
Dairy	
Protein	
Fats/Sweets	
Beverages	
Comments	
Snack	
Dinner	
Grains/Starches	
Vegetables	
Fruits	
Dairy	
Protein	
Fats/Sweets	
Beverages	
Comments	

*Affirm * Confirm * Claim Your Life!*

Daily Food Diary for :_____

Food Group	Food Name and Amount
Breakfast	
Grains/Starches	
Vegetables	
Fruits	
Dairy	
Protein	
Fats/Sweets	
Beverages	
Comments	
Snack	
Lunch	
Grains/Starches	
Vegetables	
Fruits	
Dairy	
Protein	
Fats/Sweets	
Beverages	
Comments	
Snack	
Dinner	
Grains/Starches	
Vegetables	
Fruits	
Dairy	
Protein	
Fats/Sweets	
Beverages	
Comments	

Affirm * Confirm * Claim Your Life!

Daily Food Diary for :_____

Food Group	Food Name and Amount
Breakfast	
Grains/Starches	
Vegetables	
Fruits	
Dairy	
Protein	
Fats/Sweets	
Beverages	
Comments	
Snack	
Lunch	
Grains/Starches	
Vegetables	
Fruits	
Dairy	
Protein	
Fats/Sweets	
Beverages	
Comments	
Snack	
Dinner	
Grains/Starches	
Vegetables	
Fruits	
Dairy	
Protein	
Fats/Sweets	
Beverages	
Comments	

Supreme Health & Fitness!   Knowledge Of Self Series Vol 2!

*Affirm * Confirm * Claim Your Life!*

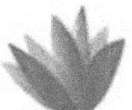 Gratitude Journal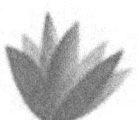

MORNING GRATITUDE PRAYER
Before you begin your day, list 10 things you're grateful for (big or small!).

1.
2.
3.
4.
5.
6.
7.
8.
9.
10.

WHAT I'M LEARNING FROM MY CHALLENGES
List 3 challenging situations, people, or other obstacles and what good thing you're learning from this challenge.

1.

I'm learning:

2.

I'm learning:

3.

I'm learning:

PEOPLE I'M THANKFUL FOR
List 5 people who made your life a little happier today. They could be friends, family, or even strangers!

1.
2.
3.
4.
5.

THE BEST PART OF MY DAY
Choose one moment of your day that made you happy and focus on it for 5 minutes before you go to sleep.

*Affirm * Confirm * Claim Your Life!*

MORNING GRATITUDE PRAYER
Before you begin your day, list 10 things you're grateful for (big or small!).

1.
2.
3.
4.
5.
6.
7.
8.
9.
10.

WHAT I'M LEARNING FROM MY CHALLENGES
List 3 challenging situations, people, or other obstacles and what good thing you're learning from this challenge.

1.

I'm learning:

2.

I'm learning:

3.

I'm learning:

PEOPLE I'M THANKFUL FOR
List 5 people who made your life a little happier today. They could be friends, family, or even strangers!

1.
2.
3.
4.
5.

THE BEST PART OF MY DAY
Choose one moment of your day that made you happy and focus on it for 5 minutes before you go to sleep.

*Affirm * Confirm * Claim Your Life!*

MORNING GRATITUDE PRAYER
Before you begin your day, list 10 things you're grateful for (big or small!).

1.
2.
3.
4.
5.
6.
7.
8.
9.
10.

WHAT I'M LEARNING FROM MY CHALLENGES
List 3 challenging situations, people, or other obstacles and what good thing you're learning from this challenge.

1.

I'm learning:

2.

I'm learning:

3.

I'm learning:

PEOPLE I'M THANKFUL FOR
List 5 people who made your life a little happier today. They could be friends, family, or even strangers!

1.
2.
3.
4.
5.

THE BEST PART OF MY DAY
Choose one moment of your day that made you happy and focus on it for 5 minutes before you go to sleep.

Affirm * Confirm * Claim Your Life!

MORNING GRATITUDE PRAYER
Before you begin your day, list 10 things you're grateful for (big or small!).

1.
2.
3.
4.
5.
6.
7.
8.
9.
10.

WHAT I'M LEARNING FROM MY CHALLENGES
List 3 challenging situations, people, or other obstacles and what good thing you're learning from this challenge.

1.

I'm learning:

2.

I'm learning:

3.

I'm learning:

PEOPLE I'M THANKFUL FOR
List 5 people who made your life a little happier today. They could be friends, family, or even strangers!

1.
2.
3.
4.
5.

THE BEST PART OF MY DAY
Choose one moment of your day that made you happy and focus on it for 5 minutes before you go to sleep.

Supreme Health & Fitness!　　　　　　　　　　Knowledge Of Self Series Vol 2!

Affirm * Confirm * Claim Your Life!

Challenging Negative Thoughts

Automatic negative thoughts (ANTs) only have power to affect our mood and lives if we let them. Sometimes ANTs can make things seem like a bigger deal than they really are, and those negative thoughts can affect the way you perceive and react to the situation. It is important to know how to control ANTs so they do not control you. Next time you feel a negative emotion and feel yourself about to react, consider these questions:

What happened?
_____
_____

Why is this upsetting?
_____
_____

What is the negative thought? How does it make you feel?
_____
_____

How does what happened affect the next 5 minutes? 24 hours? 7 days?
_____
_____

How does what happened affect your quality of life?
_____
_____

How much power are you giving the negative thought?
_____
_____

Does that negative thought deserve the control it has over you?
_____
_____

Next time you have this negative thought, what will you remind yourself to stay in control?
_____
_____

*Affirm * Confirm * Claim Your Life!*

Challenging Negative Thoughts

Automatic negative thoughts (ANTs) only have power to affect our mood and lives if we let them. Sometimes ANTs can make things seem like a bigger deal than they really are, and those negative thoughts can affect the way you perceive and react to the situation. It is important to know how to control ANTs so they do not control you. Next time you feel a negative emotion and feel yourself about to react, consider these questions:

What happened?

_____
_____

Why is this upsetting?

_____
_____

What is the negative thought? How does it make you feel?

_____
_____

How does what happened affect the next 5 minutes? 24 hours? 7 days?

_____
_____

How does what happened affect your quality of life?

_____
_____

How much power are you giving the negative thought?

_____
_____

Does that negative thought deserve the control it has over you?

_____
_____

Next time you have this negative thought, what will you remind yourself to stay in control?

_____
_____

*Affirm * Confirm * Claim Your Life!*

Challenging Negative Thoughts

Automatic negative thoughts (ANTs) only have power to affect our mood and lives if we let them. Sometimes ANTs can make things seem like a bigger deal than they really are, and those negative thoughts can affect the way you perceive and react to the situation. It is important to know how to control ANTs so they do not control you. Next time you feel a negative emotion and feel yourself about to react, consider these questions:

What happened?
_____
_____

Why is this upsetting?
_____
_____

What is the negative thought? How does it make you feel?
_____
_____

How does what happened affect the next 5 minutes? 24 hours? 7 days?
_____
_____

How does what happened affect your quality of life?
_____
_____

How much power are you giving the negative thought?
_____
_____

Does that negative thought deserve the control it has over you?
_____
_____

Next time you have this negative thought, what will you remind yourself to stay in control?
_____
_____

*Affirm * Confirm * Claim Your Life!*

Challenging Negative Thoughts

Automatic negative thoughts (ANTs) only have power to affect our mood and lives if we let them. Sometimes ANTs can make things seem like a bigger deal than they really are, and those negative thoughts can affect the way you perceive and react to the situation. It is important to know how to control ANTs so they do not control you. Next time you feel a negative emotion and feel yourself about to react, consider these questions:

What happened?
_____
_____

Why is this upsetting?
_____
_____

What is the negative thought? How does it make you feel?
_____
_____

How does what happened affect the next 5 minutes? 24 hours? 7 days?
_____
_____

How does what happened affect your quality of life?
_____
_____

How much power are you giving the negative thought?
_____
_____

Does that negative thought deserve the control it has over you?
_____
_____

Next time you have this negative thought, what will you remind yourself to stay in control?
_____
_____

*Affirm * Confirm * Claim Your Life!*

Building Self Esteem

Month _____

	1	2	3	4	5	6	7	8	9	10	11	12	13	14	15	16	17	18	19	20	21	22	23	24	25	26	27	28	29	30	31
ACHIEVEMENTS																															
Today I helped someone else																															
Today I learned something new																															
Did something I enjoy doing																															
Received a compliment																															
Tried something outside of my comfort zone																															
Did something new																															
SELF CARE																															
Took care of personal hygiene																															
Exercised																															
Ate healthy foods																															
Today I dressed in clothes that made me feel good																															
Went outdoors																															
GOALS																															
Set a realistic goal																															
Took small step toward goal																															
Reached a goal																															
RELATIONSHIPS																															
Avoided person that makes me feel bad about myself																															
Placed my needs first																															
Protected self from an unsafe person																															
You said "No"																															

Supreme Health & Fitness! *Knowledge Of Self Series Vol 2!*

*Affirm * Confirm * Claim Your Life!*

Building Self Esteem

Month _____

	1	2	3	4	5	6	7	8	9	10	11	12	13	14	15	16	17	18	19	20	21	22	23	24	25	26	27	28	29	30	31
ACHIEVEMENTS																															
Today I helped someone else																															
Today I learned something new																															
Did something I enjoy doing																															
Received a compliment																															
Tried something outside of my comfort zone																															
Did something new																															
SELF CARE																															
Took care of personal hygiene																															
Exercised																															
Ate healthy foods																															
Today I dressed in clothes that made me feel good																															
Went outdoors																															
GOALS																															
Set a realistic goal																															
Took small step toward goal																															
Reached a goal																															
RELATIONSHIPS																															
Avoided person that makes me feel bad about myself																															
Placed my needs first																															
Protected self from an unsafe person																															
You said "No"																															

*Affirm * Confirm * Claim Your Life!*

Building Self Esteem

Month _____

	1	2	3	4	5	6	7	8	9	10	11	12	13	14	15	16	17	18	19	20	21	22	23	24	25	26	27	28	29	30	31
ACHIEVEMENTS																															
Today I helped someone else																															
Today I learned something new																															
Did something I enjoy doing																															
Received a compliment																															
Tried something outside of my comfort zone																															
Did something new																															
SELF CARE																															
Took care of personal hygiene																															
Exercised																															
Ate healthy foods																															
Today I dressed in clothes that made me feel good																															
Went outdoors																															
GOALS																															
Set a realistic goal																															
Took small step toward goal																															
Reached a goal																															
RELATIONSHIPS																															
Avoided person that makes me feel bad about myself																															
Placed my needs first																															
Protected self from an unsafe person																															
You said "No"																															

Supreme Health & Fitness! Knowledge Of Self Series Vol 2!

*Affirm * Confirm * Claim Your Life!*

Building Self Esteem

Month _____

	1	2	3	4	5	6	7	8	9	10	11	12	13	14	15	16	17	18	19	20	21	22	23	24	25	26	27	28	29	30	31
ACHIEVEMENTS																															
Today I helped someone else																															
Today I learned something new																															
Did something I enjoy doing																															
Received a compliment																															
Tried something outside of my comfort zone																															
Did something new																															
SELF CARE																															
Took care of personal hygiene																															
Exercised																															
Ate healthy foods																															
Today I dressed in clothes that made me feel good																															
Went outdoors																															
GOALS																															
Set a realistic goal																															
Took small step toward goal																															
Reached a goal																															
RELATIONSHIPS																															
Avoided person that makes me feel bad about myself																															
Placed my needs first																															
Protected self from an unsafe person																															
You said "No"																															

*Affirm * Confirm * Claim Your Life!*

Building Self Esteem

Month _____

	1	2	3	4	5	6	7	8	9	10	11	12	13	14	15	16	17	18	19	20	21	22	23	24	25	26	27	28	29	30	31
ACHIEVEMENTS																															
Today I helped someone else																															
Today I learned something new																															
Did something I enjoy doing																															
Received a compliment																															
Tried something outside of my comfort zone																															
Did something new																															
SELF CARE																															
Took care of personal hygiene																															
Exercised																															
Ate healthy foods																															
Today I dressed in clothes that made me feel good																															
Went outdoors																															
GOALS																															
Set a realistic goal																															
Took small step toward goal																															
Reached a goal																															
RELATIONSHIPS																															
Avoided person that makes me feel bad about myself																															
Placed my needs first																															
Protected self from an unsafe person																															
You said "No"																															

Supreme Health & Fitness! Knowledge Of Self Series Vol 2!

Affirm * Confirm * Claim Your Life!

Resources & References

Julie Dirksen, *Design for How People Learn.* New Riders, 2012.

Mariale Hardiman, *Neuroeducation: Learning, Arts, and the Brain.* Dana Foundation, 2009.

Christina Hinton, Kurt W. Fischer, and Catherine Glennon, *Mind, Brain, and Education.* Jobs for the Future, 2012.

Mary Helen Immordino-Yang and Antonio Damasio, "We Feel, Therefore We Learn: The Relevance of Affective and Social Neuroscience to Education." *Mind, Brain, and Education,* March 2007.

Organization for Economic Corporation and Development, *Understanding the Brain: The Birth of a Learning Science.* OECD Publishing, 2007.

Affirm * Confirm * Claim Your Life!

www.ingramcontent.com/pod-product-compliance
Lightning Source LLC
Chambersburg PA
CBHW080955170526
45158CB00010B/2810